Statins
in General Practice

Statins
in General Practice

Allan Gaw, MD, PhD

Director, Clinical Trials Unit
Glasgow Royal Infirmary
Glasgow G4 0SF
UK

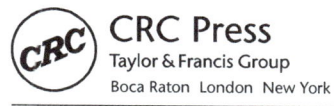

CRC Press
Taylor & Francis Group
Boca Raton London New York

CRC Press is an imprint of the
Taylor & Francis Group, an **informa** business

CRC Press
Taylor & Francis Group
6000 Broken Sound Parkway NW, Suite 300
Boca Raton, FL 33487-2742

International Standard Book Number: 978-1-8418-4349-0 (pbk)

**Library of Congress Cataloging-in-Publication Data and
The British Library Cataloging in Publication Data are Available**

**Visit the Taylor & Francis Web site at
http://www.taylorandfrancis.com**

**and the CRC Press Web site at
http://www.crcpress.com**

Statins
in General Practice

Allan Gaw, MD, PhD

Director, Clinical Trials Unit
Glasgow Royal Infirmary
Glasgow G4 0SF
UK

Supported by an educational grant from
Bristol-Myers Squibb and Sankyo Pharma UK Ltd

© 2001 Martin Dunitz Ltd, a member of the Taylor & Francis group

First published in the United Kingdom in 2001 by Martin Dunitz Ltd,
The Livery House, 7–9 Pratt Street, London NW1 0AE

Tel.:   +44 (0)20 7482 2202
Fax: +44 (0)20 7267 0159
E-mail: info.dunitz@tandf.co.uk
Website: http://www.dunitz.co.uk

A CIP record for this book is available from the British Library.

ISBN 1-84184-117-X

Distributed in the USA by
Fulfilment Center
Taylor & Francis
7625 Empire Drive
Florence, KY 41042, USA
Toll Free Tel: 1-800-634-7064
Email: cserve@routledge_ny.com

Distributed in Canada by
Taylor & Francis
74 Rolark Drive
Scarborough
Ontario M1R G2, Canada
Toll Free Tel: 1-877-226-2237
Email: tal_fran@istar.ca

Distributed in the rest of the world by
ITPS Limited
Cheriton House
North Way, Andover
Hampshire SP10 5BE, UK
Tel: +44 (0) 1264 332424
Email: reception@itps.co.uk

Printed and bound in Italy by Printer Trento S.r.l.

Contents

Allan Gaw, MD, PhD

Dr Gaw is currently Director of the Clinical Trials Unit at Glasgow Royal Infirmary and is responsible for the conduct of major clinical trials in the lipid and hypertension fields. He has been researching the pharmacology and clinical effectiveness of statins for more than a decade and has lectured widely to general practitioners and practice nurses on the use of statins in primary care. He is the author of *Clinical Biochemistry: An Illustrated Colour Text* (Churchill Livingstone, 1995), *Coronary Risk Factors: Measurement and Management* (Martin Dunitz, 1999) and co-editor of *Coronary Heart Disease Prevention: A Handbook for the Healthcare Team* (Churchill Livingstone, 1997), and *Statins: The HMG CoA Reductase Inhibitors in Perspective* (Martin Dunitz, 2000).

Disclaimer

Although every attempt has been made to provide accurate and up to date prescribing information, this is an evolving field and the prescriber should always check the most recent data sheet for the latest details of each drug mentioned.

Preface

After a long period of doubt and confusion the use of statins in clinical practice has now become an established part of modern medical care. The statins were introduced in the late 1980s and early 1990s as a new group of cholesterol-lowering drugs in an attempt to offer patients with hypercholesterolaemia a safe and effective means of reducing their plasma cholesterol. This they achieved and clinicians began to use them in place of alternative therapies such as sequestrant resins and fibrates even before the publication of the large intervention studies. But it was with the startling results of studies such as 4S, WOSCOPS, CARE and LIPID that the statins came to be thought of in a different light. From simple, but highly effective, cholesterol-lowering drugs the statins are now regarded as drugs that have an important effect in reducing not only blood lipid levels but also, more importantly, an individual's risk of vascular disease.

My aim in this book is to place the use of statins in primary care in a clinical context and to explain how these remarkable drugs work. As a necessary prerequisite we will remind ourselves of the link between blood lipids and atherosclerotic disease and the nature of the disease we are trying to prevent. The pharmacology of the statins will be discussed and their comparative mechanisms explored, but practical considerations will be at the forefront throughout. Day to day problems such as deciding who should receive statin therapy will be examined in depth. Finally, we shall look into the future to see how we may use statins in the years ahead.

This book is not intended as a definitive work on the pharmacology of the statins – that can be found elsewhere. Rather, this small volume is intended to be of practical use to the members of the primary care team who, on a daily basis, are faced with prescribing and management decisions.

Every piece of writing takes time – time that could have been spent on other things and with other people. I would therefore like to acknowledge the people who were short-changed by this project – my wife Moira and our children, Stephen and Alexandra. Without their forgiveness this work could not have been finished.

Allan Gaw

1   Why do we use statins?

Over the past 25 years, enormous resources have been put into the study of human lipid and lipoprotein metabolism. Similarly, great efforts have been made to develop and test drugs that alter the lipid profile. The reason for these endeavours is simple. We now know that a raised blood cholesterol concentration causes atherosclerosis. This disease process in turn causes coronary, cerebral and peripheral vascular disease and, by lowering the blood cholesterol level, we can prevent a significant proportion of these diseases. This book focuses specifically on the statins, a group of drugs that indisputably have had the most important impact in this field.

It is important, however, to remember that when we prescribe statins we do so in an attempt to reduce the risk of vascular disease in our patients and not simply to lower cholesterol. Cholesterol lowering has been the focus of much of our attention over the years, but cholesterol lowering per se is not our primary goal – it is to prevent heart attacks and strokes in our at-risk patients.

Because of this, it is a necessary prerequisite to understand the nature of the disease that we are targetting before we go on to consider the statins themselves.

Risk factors for CHD

There are now a large number of characteristics or traits that have been identified as risk factors for coronary heart disease (CHD). A small number of these function as independent risk factors, that is they exert their influence independent of the presence of any other risk factor. There are many others that are secondary, that is they have a positive correlation with CHD but require the presence of other risk factors for this to be manifest. It is useful to consider risk factors in the clinical setting as those which can be modified, either by lifestyle changes or therapeutic intervention, and those which are not modifiable. A list of the major risk factors is shown in Table 1.1.

It is important to realize that risk factors do not generally occur in isolation but tend to cluster in an individual. This is significant because when risk factors coexist they interact and their combined effect is much greater than would be expected from the sum of their individual effects.

The concept of multiple CHD risk factors is of great practical importance because it means that the patient at greatest risk is not necessarily the individual with a single serious risk factor such as severe hypercholesterolaemia. Instead, the individual with a poor profile of risk factors, such as the male smoker with moderate hypertension and moderately elevated lipids, is at relatively greater risk. This is illustrated in Figure 1.1.

While this book focuses on hyperlipidaemia as a risk factor for vascular disease, it is important to recognize that other risk factors are equally important. In clinical terms any attempt to modify a patient's vascular disease risk profile must attend to all the major correctable risk factors especially dyslipidaemia, smoking and hypertension.

Table 1.1   Risk factors for CHD.

Modifiable	Non-modifiable
Smoking	Age
Raised blood pressure	Male sex
Raised LDL cholesterol	Family history of CHD
Low HDL cholesterol	Personal history of CHD
Raised triglyceride	
Diabetes mellitus	
Obesity	
Diet	
Thrombogenic factors	
Lack of exercise	
Excessive alcohol consumption	

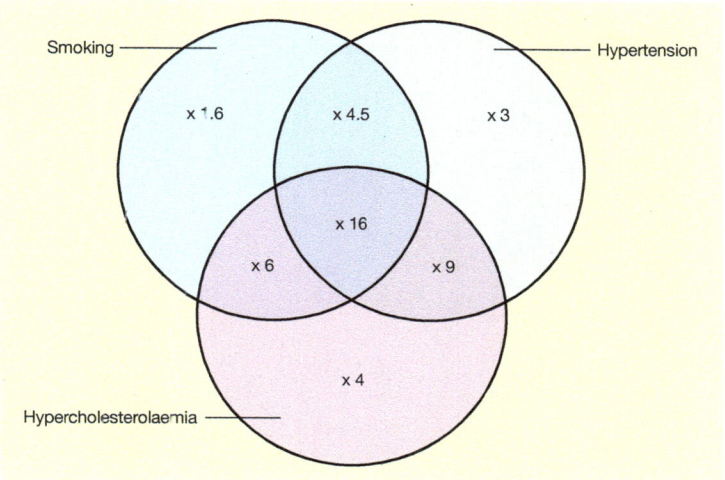

Figure 1.1   Levels of risk associated with smoking, hypertension and hypercholesterolaemia. (Adapted from Poulter et al, 1993.)

Dyslipidaemia

Cholesterol and LDL

The identification of cholesterol as a possible risk factor for CHD was first made after the recognition that in countries with a high mean blood cholesterol the mortality from CHD was also high. Figure 1.2 shows the results from one such study which illustrates the relationship between mean total cholesterol and number of CHD deaths. The country with the highest cholesterol levels in this study, Finland, also experienced the highest CHD mortality.

The position of Japan on this graph is significant as it experiences a relatively low CHD mortality. This is in keeping with the generally low cholesterol levels of the Japanese, but occurs in spite of high population rates of smoking and hypertension, two other important risk factors for CHD. This relationship has been studied further in the Ni-Hon-San study, which looked at CHD rates and risk factors in Japanese men in three societies. The results of this are summarized

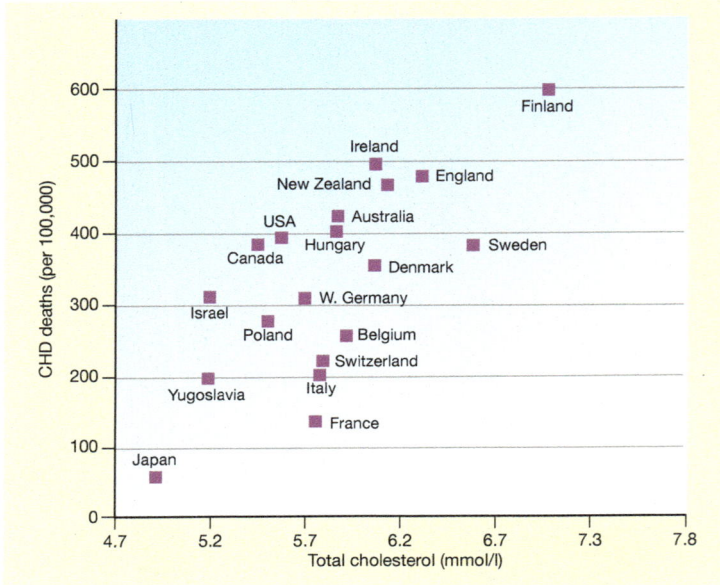

Figure 1.2   International relationship between CHD mortality and total serum cholesterol. (Adapted from Simons, 1986.)

in Table 1.2. It is clear from this that serum cholesterol level is one of the most important factors in predicting CHD risk in the population.

Cholesterol is directly involved in atherogenesis and it has been shown that the severity of atherosclerosis is directly proportional to the concentration of cholesterol in the blood. It is clear that diet is important as studies such as the Seven Countries Study have shown

Table 1.2   Ni-Hon-San study: CHD rates and risk factors in Japanese men in three societies. (Marmot et al, 1975.)

	Japan	Hawaii	California
Acute MI rate/1000	7.3	13.2	31.4
Hypertensive heart disease/1000	9.3	1.4	4.6
Non-smokers (%)	26.0	57.0	64.0
Serum total cholesterol (mmol/l)	4.7	5.6	5.9

that CHD is inversely related to the ratio of polyunsaturated to saturated fats in the diet.

The above studies identified the association between CHD and cholesterol, but in order to quantify the risk it was necessary to design prospective cohort studies. The results of three such studies are illustrated in Figure 1.3.

In these studies the relationship between CHD risk and cholesterol level is curvilinear. This was reinforced by the much larger MRFIT study, which was able to show that the relationship between cholesterol and CHD was not one of threshold, that is there is a graded and continuous risk and there is probably no cholesterol level which can be considered completely safe.

There has been some concern over the risks of low cholesterol as MRFIT demonstrated a J-shaped relationship between total

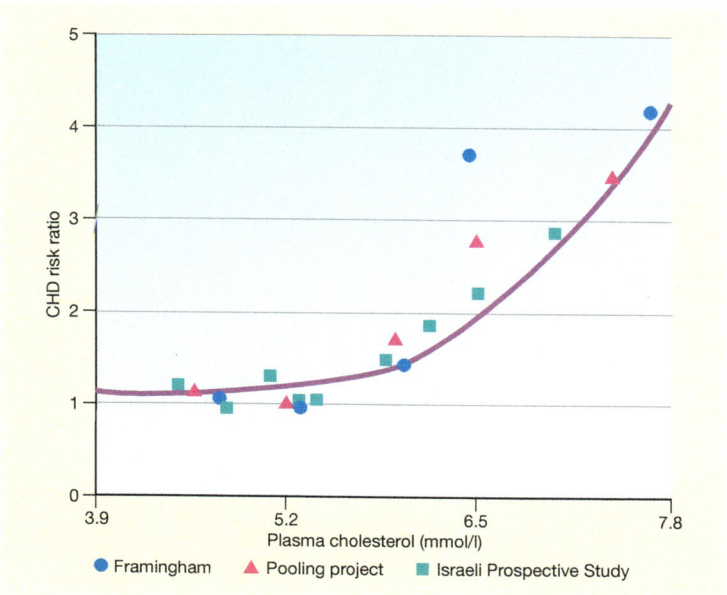

Figure 1.3   Relation between plasma cholesterol level and relative risk of CHD in three prospective studies. (Adapted from Grundy, 1986.)

cholesterol and total mortality. These relationships are compared in Figure 1.4. This increase in total mortality occurring at cholesterol levels below 4 mmol/l has been duplicated in other studies and it has been suggested that low cholesterol causes cancer. International comparative data do not support this hypothesis. For example, in Japan where 90% of men have cholesterol levels below 4.4 mmol/l the overall risk of cancer is no greater than that experienced by American or northern European men. A more likely explanation is that a low serum cholesterol is an effect of cancer rather than a cause.

Our discussion so far has centred on total cholesterol as a risk factor, but since 60–70% of plasma cholesterol is transported in the form of LDL, the effects of total cholesterol reflect the effects of LDL cholesterol.

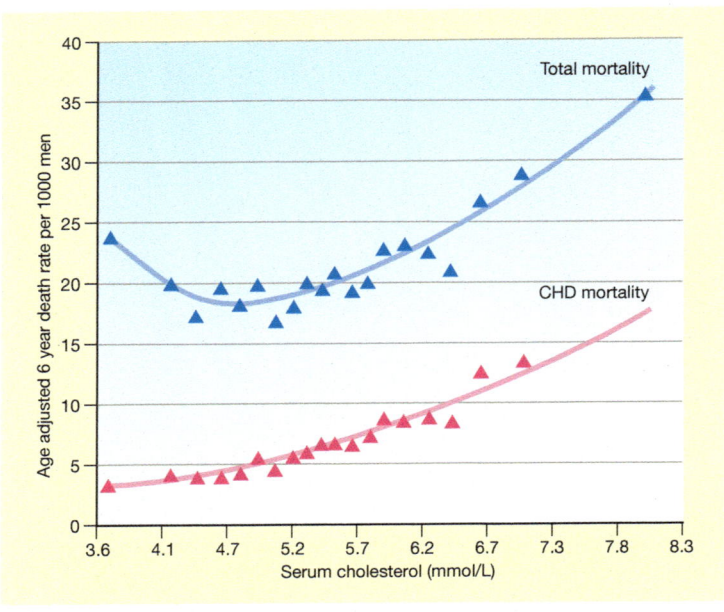

Figure 1.4   CHD and total mortality according to serum total cholesterol. (Adapted from Martin et al, 1983.)

HDL cholesterol

There is considerable evidence to support an inverse relationship between plasma HDL and CHD risk. This inverse relationship exists for both men and women and is equally strong in patients with established heart disease as well as in those who are asymptomatic. Premenopausal women have levels of HDL cholesterol which are 0.2–0.3 mmol/l higher than those of men. After the menopause this difference diminishes with increasing age and may partly explain the relative protection of women from CHD.

Plasma HDL is lowered by:

- Smoking
- Obesity
- Physical inactivity

Modification of these factors reverses the HDL-lowering effect. Diets containing high polyunsaturated fat levels have been shown to decrease LDL cholesterol while simultaneously lowering HDL, but it is possible to lower LDL cholesterol while maintaining HDL levels by reducing saturated fat and substituting moderate amounts of monounsaturated and polyunsaturated fats.

The importance of HDL as a risk factor is related to LDL levels, and the ratio of total cholesterol to HDL cholesterol is a better predictor of CHD risk than either of the variables alone. A ratio of 5 or less appears to be desirable and is of particular importance when considering treatment options for patients whose cholesterol levels are in the 5–6.5 mmol/l range.

Atherosclerosis

Atherosclerosis is a pathological process, which may be defined as a focal, inflammatory fibro-proliferative response to multiple forms of endothelial injury. The response to injury hypothesis for the development of atherosclerosis was formally proposed more than 20 years ago and has been refined and developed since.

The first lesions that may be recognized as truly atherosclerotic are called fatty streaks (Figure 1.5a). These are small lesions that, on gross inspection, are hardly raised, and are caused by localized collections of lipid-filled macrophages (foam cells) within the intima. The fatty streak lesion may be the precursor of larger atherosclerotic plaques but also may be an entirely reversible phenomenon. Such a belief comes from necropsy studies of infants from societies around the world where atherosclerosis as a cause of death is relatively rare. These infants, although unlikely to have died from CHD if they had lived to maturity, have many fatty streaks in their arteries.

Progression of a fatty streak to a larger, more complex lesion is believed to occur through two key processes. First the foam cells begin to die and break down in the centre of the fatty streak. Release of their cytoplasmic contents leads to the presence of extracellular lipids and the secretion of growth factors as part of the inflammatory response.

Smooth muscle cell migration and proliferation is the second process involved in the progression of the fatty streak (Figure 1.5b). Smooth muscle cells push into the lipid-rich plaque where they divide and begin to synthesize a connective tissue matrix. The increase in cell numbers and the laying down of collagenous matrix both serve to increase the bulk of the plaque, which now protrudes into the artery lumen and is referred to as a raised fibrolipid or advanced plaque. Such plaques are difficult to age but necropsy studies suggest that they take approximately 10–15 years to develop. It is also believed that new fatty streaks are continually forming throughout adult life.

Plaque rupture and thrombosis

The atherosclerotic plaque poses a threat to the integrity of the coronary blood flow by its size, but more importantly by its tendency to fissure and rupture. The final pathway to a major clinical event, such as an acute myocardial infarction, is not clear but rupture or fissuring of a plaque, haemorrhage into the plaque or thrombosis on its surface are all mechanisms that are likely to be involved (Figure 1.5c).

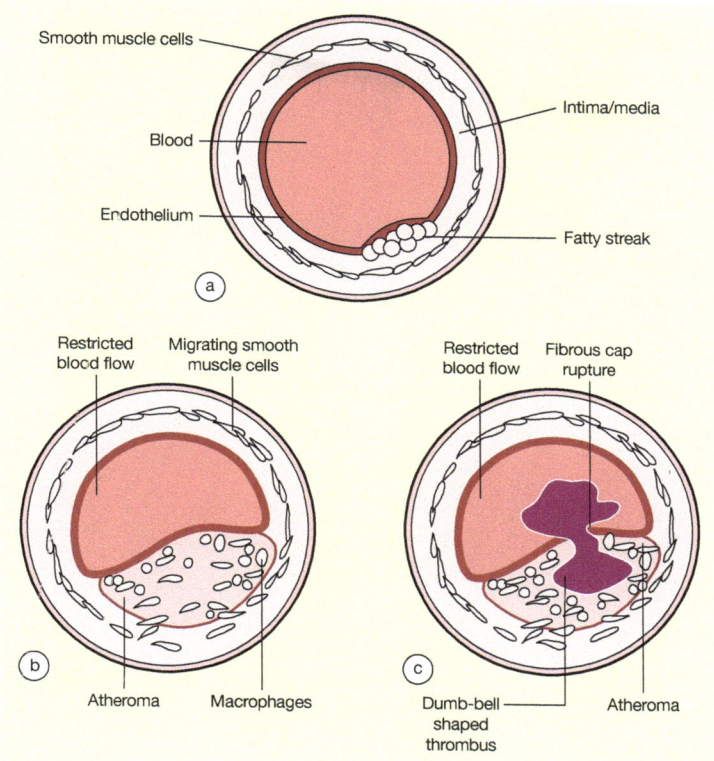

Figure 1.5   Pathogenesis of atherosclerosis. (a) As a result of endothelial injury monocytes/macrophages adhere to the endothelial surface and begin to invade the subendothelial space. By ingesting lipoproteins these cells become lipid-filled foam cells and as they accumulate at the lesion site they bulge under the endothelial surface, creating the physical appearance of the fatty streak. (b) As the lesion increases in size smooth muscle cells proliferate and migrate into the subendothelial space and platelet mural thrombi may form on the surface. The lesion may now be called an intermediate atheromatous plaque. Progression of these processes by continual release of regulatory molecules that stimulate and recruit other cells to the site and the laying down of fibrous tissue leads to the development of an advanced plaque. Note that this entire process is by no means a one way system and reversal of each of the steps is now thought to be clinically possible. (c) The plaque has a large defect in the fibrous cap, through which a dumb-bell shaped thrombus has formed, part being in the plaque and part partially occluding the lumen of the artery.

In patients with unstable angina and acute myocardial infarction it has been shown that thrombus formation is an important and dynamic process. Post-mortem studies have shown that coronary thrombi are nearly all related to the fissuring of the atheromatous plaque. The factors which determine whether thrombus does occur within the lumen are partially local, including the size and geometry of the intimal tear, whether lipid is extruded into the lumen itself, the degree of stenosis and blood flow rate at the site. Systemic factors such as the thrombotic or thrombolytic potential at the time will also play a part.

Regression of the atherosclerotic plaque

The concept of therapeutic intervention producing reversal or regression of atherosclerotic lesions originates 50 years ago when post-mortem examinations on individuals who had suffered great weight losses prior to their death revealed that the extent of plaque development in the aorta and coronary arteries was much less than expected.

That regression is possible clinically has since been proven in randomized, controlled clinical studies using lipid-lowering therapy. In the Familial Atherosclerosis Treatment Study, middle-aged men who had moderately elevated LDL, a family history of CHD and angiographic evidence of CHD had reduced frequency of progression of coronary lesions and increased frequency of regression and reduced incidence of CHD events if prescribed lipid-lowering therapy.

Clinical manifestations of atherosclerosis

Atherosclerosis may occur in many different arteries. The most common clinical manifestations are seen when the coronary arteries are involved and this will be discussed further below. However, atherosclerosis can also affect the peripheral arteries, resulting in leg muscle ischaemia called intermittent claudication.

The aorta is also frequently affected and although there is seldom complete occlusion of blood flow through this, the largest of our arteries, there can be serious clinical consequences. The atherosclerotic lesions weaken the aortic wall and can contribute to the development of aneurysms, particularly in the abdominal aorta. Rupture of an aortic aneurysm will result in sudden death.

When the cerebral arteries are affected by atherosclerosis the patient may suffer a spectrum of effects ranging from mild neurological disturbances such as reversible memory loss through transient ischaemic attacks to a fatal stroke.

Clinical picture of CHD

There are a number of clinical presentations of CHD. The most common of these are:

- Sudden death
- Myocardial infarction, which may be recognized or silent
- Angina pectoris, which may be stable or unstable

Acute myocardial infarction (MI) develops when myocardial ischaemia occurs for sufficient time to cause necrosis of a localized area of the myocardium. The crushing, central chest pain of myocardial infarction is similar to that of angina pectoris, but results from irreversible myocardial ischaemia. The pain does not subside with rest or nitrate therapy and may last for several hours. The intensity of pain gives no indication as to the severity of the infarction. Indeed, particularly in the elderly, myocardial infarction may be 'silent' and present, not with pain, but with some other feature such as acute left ventricular failure. Up to 50% of all deaths from MI occur within 2 hours of onset, mainly as a result of dysrhythmia. The majority of these deaths occur outside hospital.

Diagnosis of CHD

As always in clinical medicine a good history is the most important aid in the diagnosis of CHD, but there are many other techniques available for the full evaluation of CHD. These include simple, non-invasive tests such as the resting or excercise electrogardiogram (ECG), and progress to invasive evaluations such as angiography and radionucleide imaging.

The diagnosis of acute myocardial infarction is based on the combination of clinical symptoms and signs, with serial ECG changes and serum markers of myocardial damage such as the enzymes AST and CK and/or the muscle proteins, myoglobin and troponin T. Typical ECG and enzyme changes are illustrated in Figures 1.6 and 1.7.

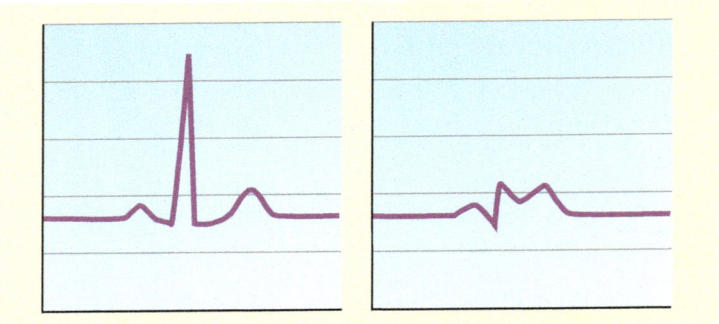

Figure 1.6   ECG changes following an MI. Left panel: normal ECG. Right panel: 2 hours after onset of chest pain. Note elevated ST segment. (Reproduced with permission from *Clinical Biochemistry: An Illustrated Colour Text*, Gaw et al, 1995.)

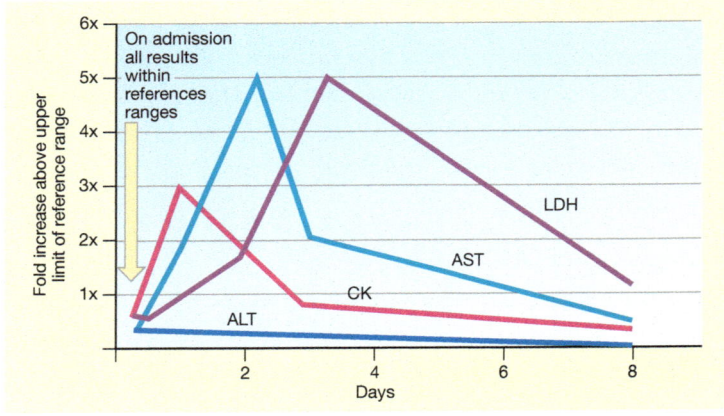

Figure 1.7   Serum enzyme changes following an uncomplicated myocardial infarction. (Reproduced with permission from *Clinical Biochemistry: An Illustrated Colour Text*, Gaw et al, 1995.)

2 How do we assess dyslipidaemia?

Lipid profiles

The most common aberrant lipid profile linked with atherogenesis and an increased risk of vascular disease is an elevated plasma LDL cholesterol level, but increasingly it is being recognized that individuals with low plasma HDL cholesterol and hypertriglyceridaemia are also at increased risk.

The units used for cholesterol and triglyceride are either mg/dl or mmol/l. The conversion factors for these are:

$$\text{Cholesterol mg/dl} = \text{mmol/l} \times 38.67$$
$$\text{Triglyceride mg/dl} = \text{mmol/l} \times 88.57$$

Blood for lipid analysis may be collected into plain containers, which will give the serum level, or into containers with the anticoagulant ethylene diamine tetra-acetic acid (EDTA), which will allow plasma levels to be measured. Tubes containing heparin should not be used. Some laboratories prefer to measure plasma levels, the advantage being that the EDTA enhances lipoprotein stability during storage; furthermore the buffy white coats of the white cells can be kept for subsequent DNA analysis. Samples may be kept for up to 4 days prior to analysis provided they are refrigerated at 4°C.

A range of different analyses may be performed on the blood sample by the biochemistry laboratory, increasing in complexity from a simple total cholesterol measurement to a full lipoprotein analysis and perhaps even DNA analysis. Most commonly, total cholesterol and triglyceride will be measured and, in addition, an HDL cholesterol level may be provided. As well as these measured values, the LDL cholesterol may be calculated, provided these three other parameters are known.

The accuracy with which the LDL cholesterol is estimated using this formula is relatively poor due to the summation of different analytical errors, but it does provide some useful information. It is important to note, however, that the Friedewald formula should not be used if the plasma triglyceride is greater than 4.0 mmol/l.

The most comprehensive (and expensive) analysis is known as a beta quantification where the total cholesterol, triglyceride, VLDL cholesterol, LDL cholesterol and HDL cholesterol will be provided. In most circumstances this full lipoprotein profile is not necessary and patients can be adequately managed with a total cholesterol, triglyceride and HDL cholesterol, with or without a calculated LDL.

Timing of samples: when to measure

If a total cholesterol measurement is all that is required then fasting is not necessary. For plasma triglyceride or lipoprotein cholesterol levels to be measured accurately the patient should have been instructed to fast. It is very important to give explicit instructions regarding fasting to ensure that the patient neither eats nor drinks anything, except water, for 12 hours prior to the blood sampling.

As with all blood chemistries there are a number of factors that affect the results of plasma lipid levels reported from the biochemistry lab:

- Biological variation which might give different results from one day to the next;
- Analytical imprecision which may produce slightly different values even if the same blood sample is measured in the same lab but on different days.

Because of these sources of variation, it is important to obtain more than one sample for lipid analysis before any action is taken. International guidelines often recommend that at least three measurements should be carried out on three separate samples before management decisions are made.

Interpretation of results

There is probably no level of cholesterol below which an individual is completely safe from the development of vascular disease. However, it is still useful to have an idea of the statistically normal range of lipid measurements which occur in the population, as the people who exist at the upper limit of these distributions are prime candidates for risk factor modification. The results obtained by the Lipid Research Council in their prevalence study to ascertain the distribution of various lipid and lipoprotein levels are shown in Table 2.1. The influence of age is clearly demonstrated here.

Table 2.1   Plasma lipid levels in American white males.

	Age (years)	Mean level (mmol/l)	5th–95th percentiles (mmol/l)
Total cholesterol	0–19	4.0	3.0–5.2
	20–24	4.3	3.2–5.4
	25–29	4.7	3.5–6.3
	30–34	4.9	3.6–6.6
	35–39	5.2	3.7–7.0
	40–44	5.3	3.9–7.0
	45–69	5.6	4.0–7.1
	70+	5.3	3.9–7.0
Triglyceride	0–9	0.6	0.3–1.1
	10–14	0.7	0.3–1.4
	15–19	0.9	0.4–1.6
	20–24	1.1	0.5–2.3
	25–29	1.3	0.5–2.8
	30–34	1.5	0.5–3.0
	35–39	1.7	0.6–3.6
	40–54	1.7	0.6–3.6
	55–64	1.6	0.6–3.3
	65+	1.5	0.6–2.9

Clinical disorders of lipid metabolism

Disorders of lipoprotein metabolism are among the commonest metabolic diseases seen in clinical practice. In addition to their important role in the development of CHD, some lipid disorders have other consequences, most notably acute pancreatitis, failure to thrive in infants, neurological disorders and the development of cataracts.

There is currently no satisfactory comprehensive classification of dyslipidaemia. The simplest means of dividing them is into primary and secondary disorders.

Classification of dyslipidemia

The Fredrickson or World Health Organization classification is the most widely accepted. This classification relies on the findings of analysis of the patient's plasma, rather than genetics. It is therefore a phenotypic rather than genotypic classification. This has a number of consequences. Patients with the same underlying genetic defect may fall into different groups, or may change grouping as their disease progresses or is treated. However, the major advantage of using this classification is that it is very widely known and gives some guidance to management. It is also important to realize that the six different classes of hyperlipoproteinaemia defined in the Fredrickson classification are not equally common in the population. Types I and V are rare, while types IIa, IIb and IV are very common. Type III hyperlipoproteinemia, also known as familial dyslipoproteinaemia, is intermediate in frequency, occurring in about 1/5000 of the population.

Genetic classifications have been attempted but are becoming increasingly complex as different mutations are discovered. Some of the recognized genetic causes of hyperlipidaemia are shown in Table 2.2. Until the advent of gene therapy and/or specific substitution therapy, genetic classifications, while biologically sound, are unlikely to prove very useful in clinical practice.

Table 2.2   Some examples of specific genetic causes of hyperlipidaemia.

Disease	Genetic defect	Fredrickson	Risk
Familial hypercholesterolaemia	Reduced numbers of functional LDL receptors	IIa or IIb	Increased risk of CHD
Familial hypertriglyceridaemia	Possibly single gene defect	IV or V	? Increased risk of CHD
Familial combined hyperlipidaemia	Possibly single gene defect	IIa, IIb, IV or V	? Increased risk of CHD
Lipoprotein lipase deficiency	Reduced levels of functional lipoprotein lipase	I	Increased risk of pancreatitis

3 What are the statins and how do they work?

Discovery

The statins are a group of drugs that owes its exsitence to the considerable efforts of Japanese and American biochemists working in the 1970s. Akira Endo and his colleagues in Japan first isolated the antibiotic mevastatin from the mould *Penicillium citrinum* in 1973, and they demonstrated that this novel compound lowered serum cholesterol levels in dogs by inhibiting the rate-limiting enzyme in cholesterol biosynthesis: hepatic 3-hydroxy-3-methyl glutaryl coenzyme A (HMG CoA) reductase.

At the time no one fully appreciated the impact that this discovery would have on vascular disease prevention worldwide, and it was only after the publication of the first large statin intervention trials in the 1990s that clinicians throughout the world truly understood what a breakthrough this was.

In considering the statins we must first answer the most commonly asked question relating to these drugs – are they all the same? The answer is perhaps predictable given our now extensive knowledge of this field of pharmacology – yes and no.

Yes, statins are all the same, for by definition they are all drugs that affect the lipid profile by inhibiting the key enzyme that controls the cell's ability to make cholesterol – HMGCoA reductase. All new compounds that share this pharmacological trait irrespective of chemical structure are likely to be suffixed '-statin'.

However, in many other pharmacological respects the statins differ significantly from each other. Before exploring further the differences between the statins it is important to understand how, as enzyme inhibitors, they control the lipid profile.

Mechanism of action

When the enzyme HMG CoA reductase is inhibited and intracellular cholesterol levels fall then the hepatocyte up-regulates the LDL receptors to import more cholesterol from the plasma (Figure 3.1). In this the statins are similar to the bile acid sequestrant resins as these drugs also ultimately result in up-regulation of the cell surface LDL receptor.

Considering the similar mechanisms of action of the statins and the resins it might be expected that their effects would be additive and indeed this is the case. LDL reductions of 60% have been observed when the drugs have been used in combination.

Despite its name the LDL receptor is also involved in clearing other more triglyceride-rich lipoproteins from the plasma and as such when statins up-regulate the receptor there is also a fall in circulating triglyceride as well as LDL cholesterol. This effect on plasma triglyceride is common to all statins but the magnitude of the fall is

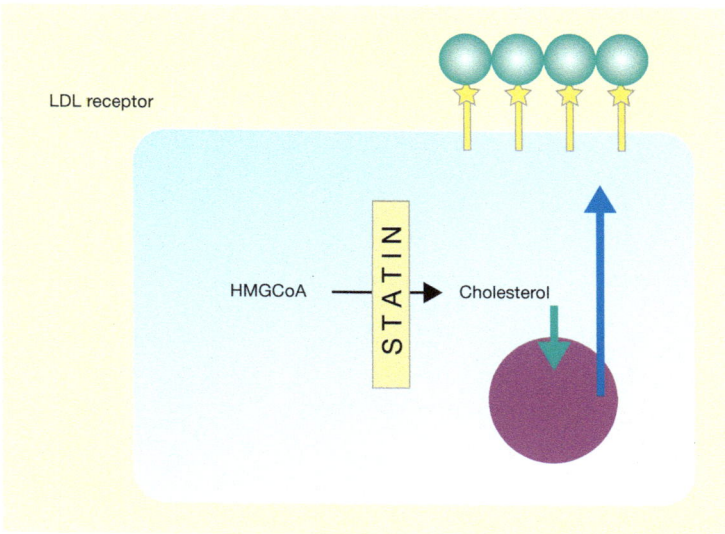

Figure 3.1   Up-regulation of the cell surface LDL receptors in response to inhibition of HMGCoA reductase by statin therapy.

proportional to the starting triglyceride level, thus those with hypertriglyceridaemia may experience 25% reductions in triglyceride and cholesterol, while normotriglyceridaemic subjects may only experience 5–10% reductions in triglyceride but greater reductions in cholesterol.

Plasma levels of HDL cholesterol are also significantly increased by statin therapy (e.g. 5–10%), although the precise mechanisms are unclear. Certainly most manoeuvres that lower plasma triglyceride also raise HDL cholesterol as the two are very closely linked metabolically.

Comparative pharmacokinetics

The structures of the statins as shown in Figure 3.2 reveal some small but important differences and these translate into pharmacokinetic differences which are shown in Table 3.1. Most notable is the fact that pravastatin is unique amongst the marketed statins to date in being water soluble, while atorvastatin has by far the greatest plasma half-life (approximately 14 hours compared to 2–3 hours for all the other statins).

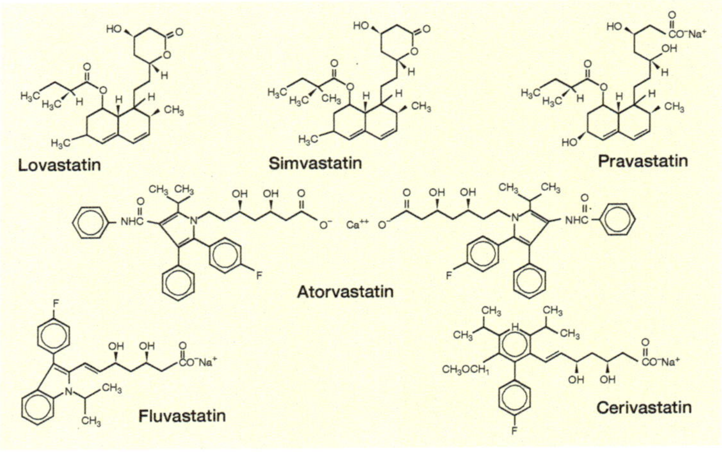

Figure 3.2   Comparative chemical structures of the statins.

Table 3.1   Comparative pharmacokinetics of the statins.

Pharmacokinetic parameter	Lovastatin	Simvastatin	Pravastatin	Fluvastatin	Atorvastatin	Cerivastatin
Major metabolic isoenzyme	3A4	3A4	None	2C9	3A4	3A4
Lipophilic	Yes	Yes	No	Yes	Yes	Yes
Protein binding (%)	>95	95–98	~50	>98	98	>99
Active metabolites	Yes	Yes	No	No	Yes	Yes
Elimination half-life (hrs)	3	2	1.8	1.2	14	2

*Not to a clinically significant extent.

Mechanism beyond cholesterol lowering

Laboratory and clinical evidence is certainly accumulating to the effect that individual statins may possess benefits beyond their cholesterol lowering capability, particularly with regard to:

- Plaque stabilization
- Endothelial function
- Cellular immunity
- Anti-inflammation
- Lipoprotein oxidation
- Rheology and blood coagulation
- Glucose intolerance

Each of these potential benefits is evaluated and summarized below.

Statins and plaque stabilization

Before the statins were introduced, clinical trial experience with earlier lipid-lowering drugs had suggested that an inevitable delay of 2 years or more was to be expected prior to the onset of benefit from cholesterol reduction. Most pathologists linked this to essential remodelling of the atherosclerotic lesion, which they imagined led to its shrinkage and, in consequence, an improvement in downstream tissue perfusion.

Large, pre-occlusive lesions were therefore considered to be the primary target for intervention strategies, consistent with the abundant experimental evidence that links the total vascular atherosclerosis burden to ultimate risk of cardiovascular death. However, despite the welcome provision of symptomatic relief, surgical intervention, in contrast to medical management of risk factors, does not extend life or reduce coronary mortality overall. This suggests that the large lesion is not necessarily the culprit leading to potentially fatal events.

In this regard, recent autopsy studies have redirected our attention to what seems to be a continuing and in general asymptomatic process of lesion rupture and healing, seen equally commonly in non-

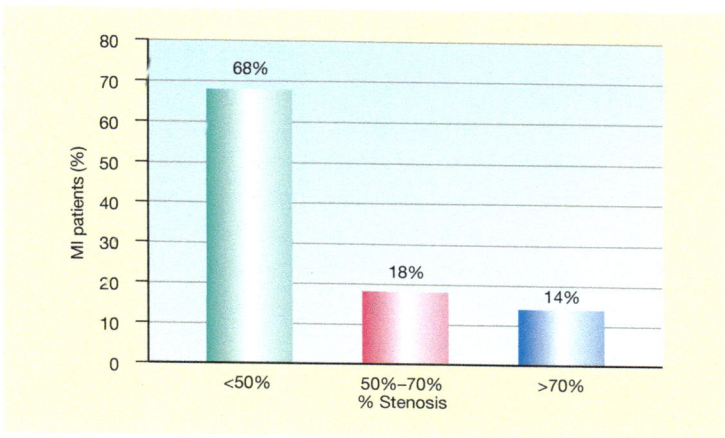

Figure 3.3   Proportion of large, medium and small atherosclerotic plaques leading to myocardial infarction. (Adapted from Falk et al, 1995.)

occlusive as in occlusive plaques (Figure 3.3). Repetition of this cycle is frequently accompanied by intramural thrombosis, leading to substantial and sudden lesion growth. Occasionally, thrombus may propagate into the vessel lumen, producing a catastrophic occlusive myocardial infarction. So, plaque vulnerability to rupture is of greater clinical relevance than plaque size. Not surprisingly, therefore, those factors which govern the vulnerability of the plaque itself are under intensive investigation. Table 3.2 describes what are thought to be the key players in this process.

Table 3.2   Characteristic features of the vulnerable atherosclerotic plaque.

Thin, fragmented fibrous cap
Underdeveloped connective tissue skeleton
Lipid enrichment
Inflammatory cell infiltration
Evidence of proteolytic enzyme release
Apoptosis

Pathological studies of patients who have died suddenly of myocardial infarction are consistent with the view that the typical causal lesion is a previously unrecognized minimally occlusive plaque, whose thin or fragmented fibrous cap, poorly supported by an underlying connective tissue skeleton, has ruptured, exposing the blood to the underlying, highly thrombogenic lipid-rich core infiltrated with inflammatory cells. Cytokines released by the latter have already attracted medial smooth muscle cells into the subintimal space. Both cell types trigger further matrix degeneration within the lesion by releasing metalloproteinases.

Statin therapy inhibits many of the above processes, helping to reduce the likelihood of plaque rupture or limiting thrombus formation should rupture occur. Comparative investigations suggest that the lipid soluble statins are capable of modulating smooth muscle cell growth, independently of their cholesterol lowering capability (Figure 3.4). Interestingly, the water soluble statin, pravastatin, has no appreciable effect on vascular smooth muscle cells at normal

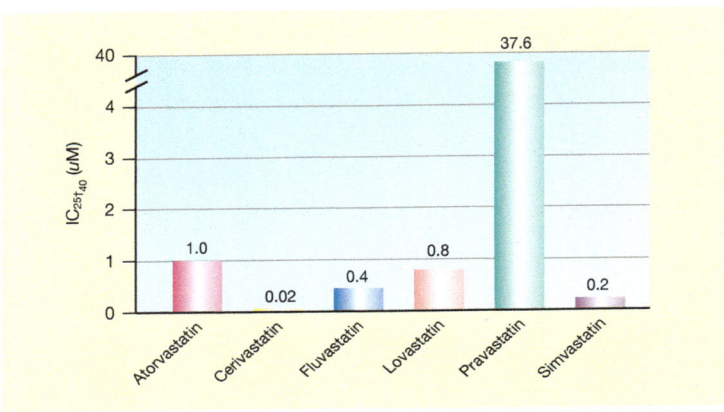

Figure 3.4   Differential effects of HMG CoA reductase inhibitors on vascular smooth muscle cells. Drug concentration required to inhibit 25% of human smooth muscle cell proliferation. Samples were obtained from the left internal mammary artery of CABG patients. Proliferation was analysed by measuring mitochondrial dehydrogenase activity. (Adapted from Soma et al, 1995.)

pharmacological doses and this is possibly explained on the basis of tissue penetration.

The statins may also exert a direct suppressant effect on platelet activation, thereby limiting platelet thrombus formation (Figure 3.5). In addition, their LDL lowering actions result in a reduction in the number of inflammatory cells within the plaque and a change in plaque

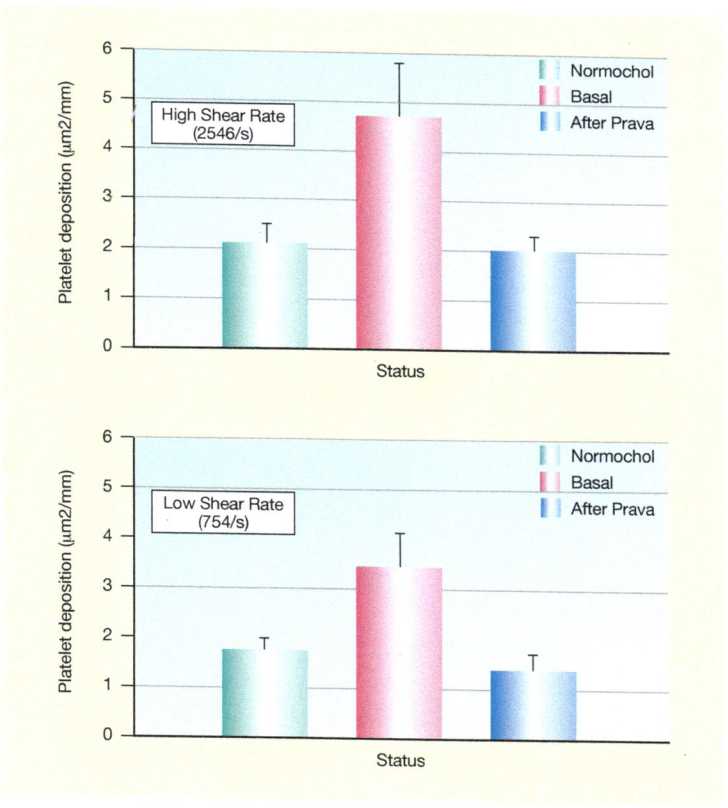

Figure 3.5   Platelet deposition and the effects of pravastatin therapy. Bar graphs showing platelet deposition at the high shear rate of 2546/s (top) and at the low shear rate of 754/s (bottom) in normocholesterolaemic (Normochol) and hypercholesterolaemic patients at baseline (Basal) and after treatment with pravastatin (After Prava). (Adapted from Lacoste et al, 1995.)

composition, leading to the development of a stiffer, more stable lesion.

Statins and endothelial function

Until relatively recently the endothelium was thought of as merely a water-tight pavement of cells lining our blood vessels, that was metabolically inactive.

This perception was challenged by the discovery that the vascular endothelium, in response to increasing flow-mediated shear stress, elaborates a chemical signal which promotes relaxation of the underlying arterial smooth muscle cells and, in consequence, coordinates vasomotor changes throughout the vascular bed. The signal is now known to be nitric oxide.

As our knowledge of this agent grows it is becoming clear that endothelium-dependent relaxation is depressed in atherosclerotic coronary arteries. Even in apparently healthy vessels, high LDL concentrations directly inhibit the relaxation process so that vasodilatation in response to acetylcholine is impaired in hypercholesterolaemia, well in advance of the structural, histologic or clinical appearance of disease. Interestingly, it appears that oxidized LDL rather than the native particle is the main culprit in this process. Hypercholesterolaemic patients seem to be unable to release nitric oxide in adequate amounts to induce vasodilatation.

Early in 1989, studies showed that the vasospasm detected in hypercholesterolaemic rabbits could be reversed or attenuated by statin therapy. These findings were soon confirmed in hypercholesterolaemic patients. Treatment with a variety of lipid lowering agents or with therapy designed to limit lipoprotein oxidation restored the physiological coronary vasodilator response to acetylcholine in proportion to the cholesterol reduction.

Statins and cellular immunity

In a prospective randomized trial of pravastatin therapy administered to heart transplant recipients the question of whether transplant vasculopathy, associated with raised plasma lipid levels, could be avoided was assessed. The surprise finding was that episodes of acute rejection were reduced and, in consequence, graft survival prolonged (Figure 3.6). This line of investigation was pursued with a second study which demonstrated prolongation of kidney graft survival following pravastatin treatment.

Several possible explanations for these intriguing findings have been proposed, including reduction in natural killer cell cytotoxicity,

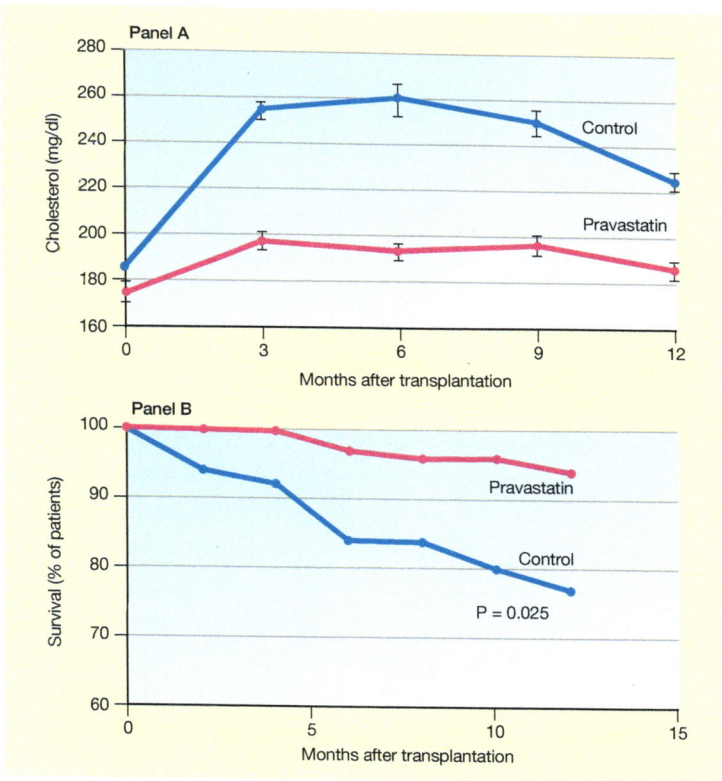

Figure 3.6   Cardiac transplant rejection and the effects of pravastatin therapy. Panel A: Mean (± SE) cholesterol levels during the first year after cardiac transplantation in the study patients (Pravastatin group n = 47, No statin n = 50). Panel B: Survival during the first year after cardiac transplantation in the study patients (Pravastatin group n = 47, No statin n = 50). (Adapted from Kobashigawa et al, 1995.)

enhancement of immunosuppression due to synergism between pravastatin and cyclosporin, and simple reduction of plasma lipid levels. In partial dismissal of the latter, it has been pointed out that the immunosuppressive action is apparently independent of the degree of cholesterol reduction achieved.

A similar effect has been demonstrated with simvastatin, but whether this effect is applicable to the whole class of HMG CoA reductase inhibitors remains to be determined. Large scale prospective clinical studies are urgently needed in this potentially very important new therapeutic use of statins.

Statins and inflammation

One of the most exciting developments in the last few years has been the appreciation that inflammatory processes play a key role in the development of the atherosclerotic plaque and that the statins may have a significant impact on these processes and therefore in the progression and destabilization of such plaques. The association between plasma levels of inflammatory markers such as C-reactive protein (CRP) and increased cardiovascular risk has been clearly demonstrated (Figure 3.7).

More recently, a subgroup of the CARE Study cohort has been examined, and CRP levels were measured at baseline and after 5 years. Among these MI survivors on standard therapy plus placebo, CRP levels tended to increase over 5 years of follow-up. In contrast, randomization to pravastatin therapy resulted in significant reductions in this inflammatory marker (-39%, $P = 0.002$) that were not related to the magnitude of lipid alterations observed. These data provide important new evidence for the non-lipid lowering effects of pravastatin and may further explain the clinical benefits seen with this drug in the large scale intervention studies, WOSCOPS, LIPID and CARE.

Statins and lipoprotein oxidation

Individuals may have raised concentrations of LDL cholesterol in their plasma because they fail to clear this lipoprotein fraction adequately

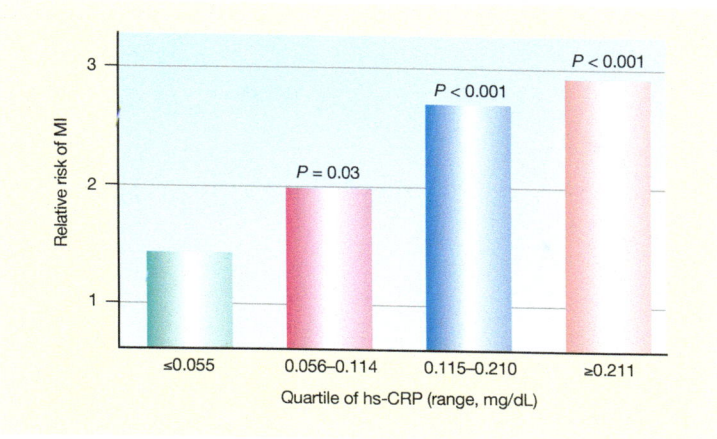

Figure 3.7   Relative risk of myocardial infarction stratified by quartile of baseline plasma CRP. (Adapted from Ridker et al, 1997.)

from their bloodstream. The circulating half-life of these particles is therefore increased and, in consequence, they are susceptible to greater levels of oxidation.

Oxidation of LDL is a prerequisite to its uptake by macrophages, a key event in early atherogenesis. Furthermore, oxidized LDL possesses additional atherogenic properties which include cytotoxicity and stimulation of thrombotic and inflammatory events.

As described above, the statins achieve their LDL lowering effect by activating the LDL receptor on the cell surface. This results in accelerated uptake of the lipoprotein by the liver and a decrease in its transit time through the plasma. The potential for lipoprotein oxidation in the circulation should consequently be reduced.

In addition to their effects on LDL metabolism, statins produce changes in the composition of the circulating lipoprotein by decreasing the cholesterol/protein ratio in the particle, in line with the concept that stimulation of hepatic LDL receptor activity results in preferential removal of cholesterol-enriched particles. Such changes again could alter the susceptibility of the lipoprotein to oxidation (Figure 3.8).

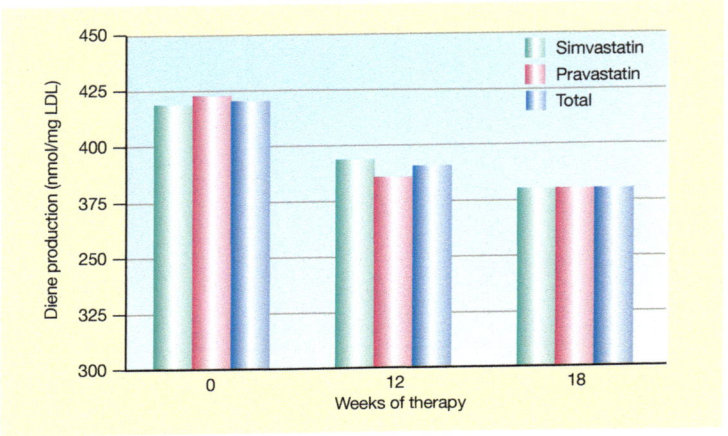

Figure 3.8   Susceptibility of LDL to in vitro oxidation and statin therapy. LDL was isolated from hypercholesterolaemic patients treated for up to 18 weeks with increasing doses of either simvastatin or pravastatin (10, 20 and 40 mg daily for 6 weeks each, respectively). $*P < 0.05$, $**P < 0.01$, $***P < 0.001$, for significance between pre- and post-treatment values. (Adapted from Kleinveld et al, 1993.)

The concept that the accelerated catabolism induced by statin therapy should reduce the age of the circulating LDL population, alter its composition and increase its resistance to oxidative modification has been tested directly in vivo. All clinically available statins were found to reduce the susceptibility of the lipoprotein to oxidation.

This decrease in lipoprotein oxidizability might be an important class-related ancillary mechanism by which statin therapy helps prevent atherosclerosis progression in man.

Statins, rheology and blood coagulation

In addition to their ability to lower plasma lipid levels, some statins also appear capable of improving platelet function and reducing blood viscosity. As illustrated in Figure 3.5, pravastatin was shown to have significant effects on platelet thrombus formation.

Similarly, statin-induced cholesterol reduction seems also to promote a fall in blood viscosity with resulting improvements in tissue perfusion. In the West of Scotland Study, treatment with pravastatin lowered plasma and whole blood viscosity (Figure 3.9). This finding was not driven by a change in plasma fibrinogen but rather by decrements in circulating LDL and VLDL.

While the magnitude of the viscosity change may appear small in numerical terms, it corresponds to the mean difference between men who suffered a myocardial infarction and those who did not, and may account for about 25% of the risk reduction achieved with pravastatin in WOSCOPS.

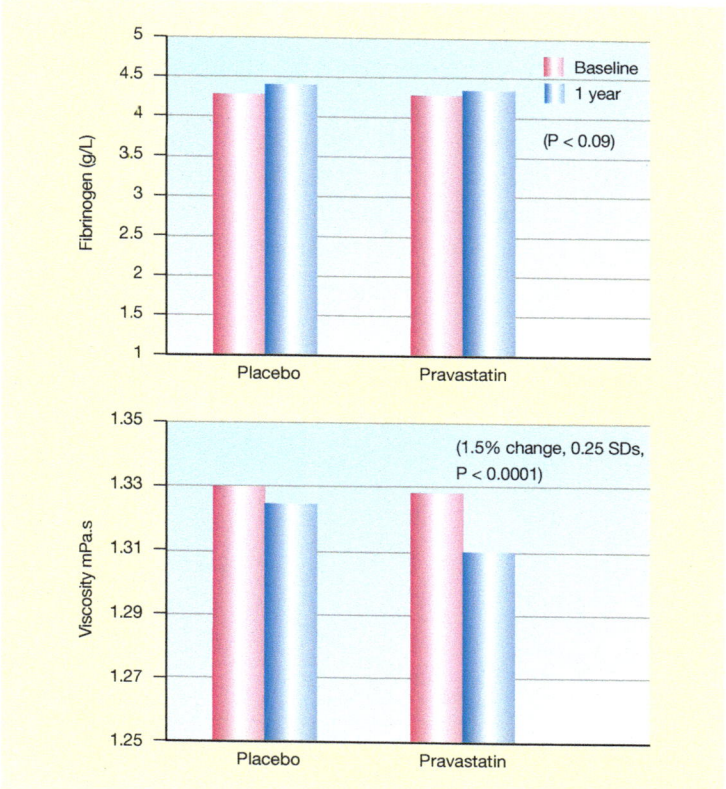

Figure 3.9   Fibrinogen and plasma viscosity and the effects of pravastatin therapy. Fibrinogen (top) and plasma viscosity (bottom) changes in the first year of WOSCOPS. (Adapted from Rumley et al, 1997.)

Statins and diabetes

In a recent analysis of the WOSCOPS study interesting new findings have emerged, which would suggest that pravastatin therapy in that cohort had a significant impact on the participants' risk of developing type 2 diabetes throughout the 5-year study.

Using a modified American Diabetes Association definition of diabetes, a total of 5940 of the 6595 randomized subjects were included in the analysis and 139 subjects became diabetic during the study. The baseline predictors of this transition to diabetes from normality were studied. Body mass index (BMI), plasma triglyceride concentration, white cell count (WCC), systolic blood pressure, total and HDL cholesterol, glucose and randomized treatment assignment to pravastatin were significant predictors.

In a multivariate model only BMI, plasma triglyceride concentration, and pravastatin therapy were predictive.

The investigators concluded that assignment to pravastatin therapy resulted in a significant reduction (30%) in the hazard of developing type 2 diabetes (Figure 3.10). Pravastatin therapy, by

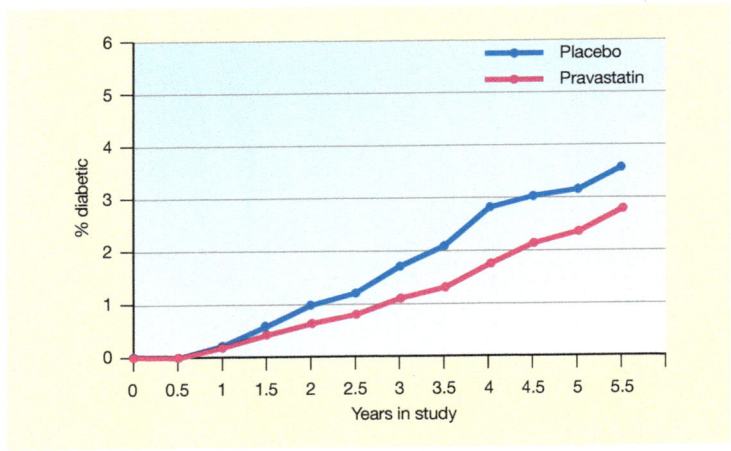

Figure 3.10   Development of diabetes in the placebo group and the pravastatin treated group in WOSCOPS.

lowering plasma triglycerides, may favourably influence the development of diabetes, but other explanations such as the anti-inflammatory properties of this drug in combination with its beneficial effects on endothelial function may prove to be important.

Clinical use

The statins are indicated in the treatment of dyslipidaemia and, following the publication of the large scale statin intervention trials outlined below, they also now have additional indications in the primary and secondary prevention of CHD.

The major contraindication to the use of statin therapy is active liver disease, although they should also be avoided in pregnancy and lactation and in women whose contraceptive methods are unreliable. Similarly, care should be taken in patients with renal impairment. None of the statins are licensed for use in children

Side effects, if they occur, are usually mild: gastrointestinal upsets, headache, fatigue and skin rashes. A much more serious side effect, namely rhabdomyolysis, has been documented but this is very rare. More commonly there may be a rise in the serum level of creatine kinase (CK or CPK). This is a marker of muscle damage and if raised by more than ten times the laboratory's upper limit of normal, the drug should be discontinued. A practical point to note, however, is that in patients of African descent the serum CK levels are normally higher than in Caucasian subjects, so the usual reference ranges may not be applicable.

Statins are available as capsules or tablets to be taken once daily, at night. The rationale for this is that cholesterol synthesis exhibits a diurnal rhythm, the maximum rate occurring at night. Since the drugs inhibit cholesterol synthesis by inhibiting the rate limiting enzyme, maximum effect should be seen if it is given at the time of peak enzyme activity. In practice, however, if a patient can be encouraged to take their statin therapy at the same time each day on a regular basis this is more important than adhering strictly to nocte dosing.

Drug–drug interactions

Because the statins are predominantly metabolized by the cytochrome P450 system in the liver there exists the possibility of drug–drug interaction at this level, because a large number of other commonly prescribed drugs are also metabolized by this system. One exception to this is pravastatin. Because of this drug's water solubility it is not metabolized to any significant extent by the liver. Theoretically, drug–drug interactions should therefore be significantly lower with pravastatin than with other statins. This may be of particular importance when patients receiving multiple other drugs are considered for statin therapy. One such group would be the elderly.

4 What evidence do we have that statins work?

We are fortunate as clinicians when it comes to statins, for over the last decade an unmatched portfolio of clinical trial results has been assembled which forms the foundation of our evidence based practice. The five largest statin studies to date are summarized in Table 4.1 and these trials will be further reviewed and summarized below.

Scandinavian Simvastatin Survival Study: 4S

This secondary prevention study, published in 1994 by the Scandinavian Survival Study Group, was a double blind, randomized,

Table 4.1   CHD prevention with statins.

Clinical trial	Drug used	Number of subjects (% male)	Relative reduction in fatal or non-fatal MI (%)
West of Scotland Coronary Prevention Study (WOSCOPS)	Pravastatin	6595 (100)	31
Cholesterol and Recurrent Events (CARE) Study	Pravastatin	4159 (86)	24
Scandinavian Simvastatin Survival Study (4S)	Simvastatin	4444 (81)	34
Long Term Intervention with Pravastatin in Ischaemic Disease (LIPID)	Pravastatin	9014 (82)	23
Air Force/Texas Coronary Prevention Study (AF/TEXCAPS)	Lovastatin	6605 (85)	36*

*Expanded endpoint of combined unstable angina, fatal and non-fatal MI and sudden cardiac death.

placebo controlled trial looking at the effects of lowering cholesterol in men and women aged between 35 and 70 who had a history of angina or myocardial infarction. The subjects recruited (4444) had cholesterol levels between 5.5 and 8.0 mmol/l and triglyceride levels less than or equal to 2.5 mmol/l. Half of the subjects were given simvastatin, 20–40 mg while the other half were given a placebo and both groups were regularly reviewed over a 5-year period.

Results

The mean changes in lipid levels observed in the simvastatin group were as follows:

- Total cholesterol fell by 25%
- LDL cholesterol fell by 35%
- Triglyceride fell by 10%
- HDL increased by 8%

The primary endpoint was total mortality and Figure 4.1 demonstrates that the mortality rates of the simvastatin and placebo groups began to diverge at around 18 months into the study and continued this trend throughout the period of the trial. From these results it was calculated that there was a 30% reduction in total mortality for the patients on simvastatin.

The secondary endpoint was major coronary events and here also there was an impressive risk reduction, of 34%, for the simvastatin treated group

The 4S study looked at two important subgroups, namely women and those over 60 years of age. The results showed that simvastatin reduced the risk of major coronary events in women to a similar extent as that seen in men and that survival rates for those over 60 years of age were significantly improved.

The study also demonstrated one important negative result: no increase in non-CHD mortality, such as death due to violence or cancer, was observed in the simvastatin group. This puts to rest suggestions made by previous studies that lowering cholesterol may lead to increased mortality from other causes.

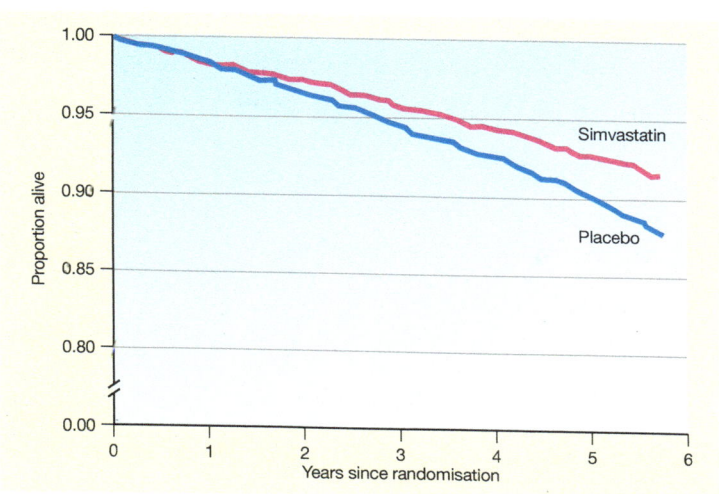

Figure 4.1   Survival curves for total mortality in 4S. (Adapted from Scandinavian Simvastatin Survival Study Group, 1994.)

The frequency of adverse events was similar for both the simvastatin and placebo groups. Rhabdomyolysis occurred in one patient on simvastatin, but recovery followed the cessation of treatment.

Overall the benefits of prescribing simvastatin to a group of 100 middle-aged, CHD patients for 6 years were summarized as follows:

- 4 of the expected 9 deaths would be avoided
- 7 of the 21 expected MIs would be prevented
- 6 out of 19 revascularization procedures would be unnecessary

West of Scotland Coronary Prevention Study: WOSCOPS

This study, published in 1995 by Shepherd and his colleagues, was of a similar design to 4S in that it was randomized, placebo controlled and double blind, but it differed in that it was concerned with primary prevention, and only men were included. A total of 6595 men, aged between 45 and 64 years with no history of myocardial infarction, were recruited. Subjects were eligible for inclusion, however, if they had stable angina, provided they had not been hospitalized over the past 12 months. LDL cholesterol levels of the participants were within the range 4.5 to 6.0 mmol/l. Recruits were given either placebo or pravastatin 40 mg to be taken in the evening.

The subjects were followed up over a 5-year period and those on pravastatin showed significant improvement in their lipid profile:

- Total cholesterol fell by 20%
- LDL cholesterol fell by 26%
- Triglyceride fell by 12%
- HDL cholesterol increased by 5%

The primary endpoint for WOSCOPS was fatal or non-fatal MI and Kaplan Meier analysis, as shown in Figure 4.2, demonstrates that this was reduced by 31%. Deaths from any cause were also reduced in the pravastatin group by 22%, and, as with 4S, there was no excess of non-cardiac deaths.

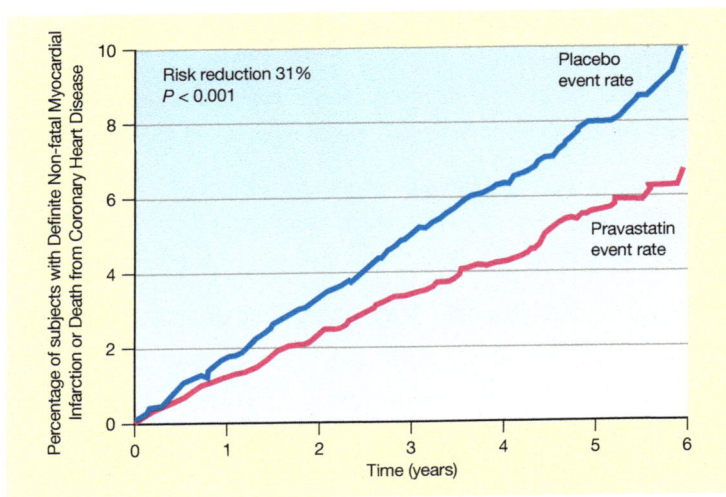

Figure 4.2   Event curve for fatal or non-fatal MI in WOSCOPS. (Adapted from Shepherd et al, 1995.)

The subgroup analysis of WOSCOPS also revealed some interesting findings. In particular, it was apparent that the benefits of pravastatin therapy were not affected by age. Those aged 55 years and older obtained the same benefit as younger subjects. Similarly, smoking habits did not counter the beneficial effect of the drug. It was also noted that a significant benefit was seen in the subgroup without multiple risk factors and in those without pre-existing vascular disease.

Extrapolation of the WOSCOPS data reveals that treatment with pravastatin over 5 years of 1000 middle-aged men with hypercholesterolaemia but with no evidence of a previous MI will avoid:

- 14 coronary angiograms
- 8 revascularization procedures
- 20 non-fatal MIs
- 7 cardiovascular deaths
- 2 deaths from other causes

Cholesterol and Recurrent Events: CARE

The CARE study was performed in multiple centres throughout the USA and Canada and was published in 1996. The objective of this secondary prevention trial was to evaluate the effects of pravastatin therapy on rates of non-fatal MI and CHD death in post-MI patients without elevated total plasma cholesterol concentrations, who continued to receive standard post-MI treatments (aspirin, beta-blockers, PTCA/CABG).

This was a double blind, placebo controlled, randomized trial of 4159 subjects aged 21–75 who were 3–20 months post-MI. The subjects in the study were randomized to receive either pravastatin (40 mg) or placebo and followed up for an average of 5 years. The primary combined endpoint was recurrent non-fatal MI or CHD death. Other endpoints of the study included coronary death, non-fatal MI, total mortality, the need for revascularization and stroke. The baseline characteristics of the study subjects are shown in Table 4.2.

Table 4.2   Characteristics of the study subjects in CARE at baseline.

	Placebo ($n = 2078$)	Pravastatin ($n = 2081$)
Mean age (years)	59	59
Total cholesterol (mg/dl)	209	209
LDL cholesterol (mg/dl)	139	139
HDL cholesterol (mg/dl)	39	39
Triglyceride (mg/dl)	155	156
% Female	14	14
% Hypertensive	43	42
% Diabetic	15	14
% Current smokers	21	21

In the CARE study pravastatin therapy resulted in:

- 32% reduction in LDL cholesterol ($P < 0.001$)
- 24% reduction in fatal or non-fatal MI ($P = 0.003$)
- 31% reduction in stroke ($P = 0.03$)
- 26% reduction in coronary artery bypass surgery (CABG) ($P = 0.005$)
- 22% reduction in coronary angioplasty (PTCA) ($P = 0.01$)

In summary, if 1000 post-MI patients with total cholesterol < 6.2 mmol/l (240 mg/dl) are treated for 5 years we would prevent 150 cardiovascular events and 51 patients would be spared from having at least one such event. For patients >60 years the corresponding figures would be 207 cardiovascular events and 71 patients. If the 1000 patients were all female the figures would be 228 cardiovascular events and 97 patients.

Air Force/Texas Coronary Atherosclerosis Prevention Study: AF/TEXCAPS

This study randomized 6605 subjects (15% women) to either placebo or lovastatin, tritrated up to 40 mg/day in order to achieve a target LDL cholesterol goal of less than 2.84 mmol/l (110 mg/dl). These individuals had no clinical evidence of atherosclerotic cardiovascular disease and the interesting feature of this study was that their baseline total plasma cholesterol level was on average 5.71 mmol/l (220 mg/dl) with an LDL cholesterol of 3.88 mmol/l (150 mg/dl). Five years of therapy changed the lipid profiles as shown below:

- Total cholesterol   −18%
- LDL cholesterol   −25%
- Triglyceride   −15%
- HDL cholesterol   +6%

Although these lipid changes did not result in significant reductions in CHD or total mortality they did result in the following significant changes:

- Combined unstable angina, fatal and non-fatal
  MI or sudden cardiac death   −37%
- Revascularizations   −33%

Long Term Intervention with Pravastatin in Ischaemic Disease: LIPID

This study revealed equally interesting data. Here, 9014 subjects (17% female) drawn from 87 centres in Australia and New Zealand and with an average total cholesterol level of 5.65 mmol/l (218 mg/dl) were randomized to pravastatin (40 mg/day) or placebo and followed for an average of 6 years. Pravastatin therapy produced the following lipid changes:

- Total cholesterol   −18%
- LDL cholesterol   −25%
- Triglyceride   −11%
- HDL cholesterol   +5%

and the following highly significant reductions in risk of mortality and morbidity:

- All cause mortality   −22%
- CHD deaths   −24%

- Fatal CHD and non-fatal MI   −24%
- Total strokes   −19%

One unique aspect of the LIPID study arose from the decision to recruit substantial numbers of patients with unstable angina. These individuals benefited in terms of event avoidance as much as recruits with a history of myocardial infarction.

In conclusion, the principal investigator of the study summarized the clinical importance of the LIPID study by stating that the results suggested, 'virtually all patients presenting with myocardial infarction or unstable angina should now be considered for drug therapy'.

Atorvastatin Versus Revascularization Treatment (AVERT) study

The Atorvastatin Versus Revascularization Treatment (AVERT) study examined the effect of aggressive lipid-lowering therapy compared with angioplasty in stable angina pectoris patients.

Three hundred and forty-one patients with stable CHD, relatively normal left ventricular function, asymptomatic or mild to moderate angina and a serum LDL cholesterol level of ≥115 mg/dl (3.0 mmol/l), referred for PTCA, were recruited. The patients were randomly assigned to either atorvastatin 80 mg/day or to undergo PTCA followed by usual care, which may include lipid lowering and even statin therapy. The follow-up period was 18 months.

Of the atorvastatin treated subjects, 13% suffered an ischaemic event compared to 21% in the angioplasty/usual care group ($P = 0.048$). Furthermore, atorvastatin treated patients had a significantly longer time to the first event compared to the control group ($P = 0.03$).

The authors concluded that in these relatively low risk patients with stable coronary disease, aggressive lipid lowering with atorvastatin therapy was at least as effective as angioplasty and usual care in reducing the incidence of ischaemic events.

Myocardial Ischaemia Reduction with Aggressive Cholesterol Lowering Study: MIRACL

The background to this study was the fact that all previous large scale statin studies had systematically excluded acute patients from recruitment. In 4S: entry >6 months post-event, in CARE: entry 3 to 20 months post-event, and in LIPID: entry 3 months to 3 years post-event. In the crucial period between the acute event and 3 months later many patients die or suffer second or subsequent events. While statin therapy has been proven to be of clinical benefit in stable patients more than 3 months after an event, no large study has examined the effects of statin therapy in this early high mortality/morbidity period.

The MIRACL study recruited 3086 patients within 24 to 96 hours of an acute coronary syndrome. They were randomized to either atorvastatin 80 mg per day or placebo for 16 weeks, both with dietary education and counselling.

Patients treated with atorvastatin experienced a significant reduction (16%, $P = 0.048$) in the risk of the primary combined endpoint of death, non-fatal MI, cardiac arrest with resuscitation or recurrent symptomatic myocardial ischaemia requiring emergency hospitalization. The reduction in this combined endpoint was primarily due to a favourable effect of atorvastatin on recurrent symptomatic myocardial ischaemia, which was reduced by 26% ($P = 0.02$). In addition, the incidence of stroke was significantly reduced in the atorvastatin treated group compared to the placebo group. Atorvastatin therapy reduced the average LDL cholesterol from 123 mg/dl (3.2 mmol/l), at baseline, to 72 mg/dl (1.9 mmol/l).

5 Who should receive statin therapy?

Evidence base

Both primary prevention and secondary prevention of CHD using statins are now based on a strong foundation of clinical trial evidence. Interestingly, the evidence gathered from the major statin trials reveals an apparently startling similarity in the clinical effectiveness of the three natural statins tested to date (simvastatin, pravastatin and lovastatin). Relative risk reductions of 25–30% in cardiovascular endpoints are seen across the trials, with virtually all patients, irrespective of baseline risk or cholesterol levels, benefitting from treatment. However, these figures do not reveal the wide variations in absolute risk reductions seen in different patient groups (Figure 5.1).

While nearly all patients benefit from statin therapy, the absolute risk reductions achieved will vary considerably depending on baseline

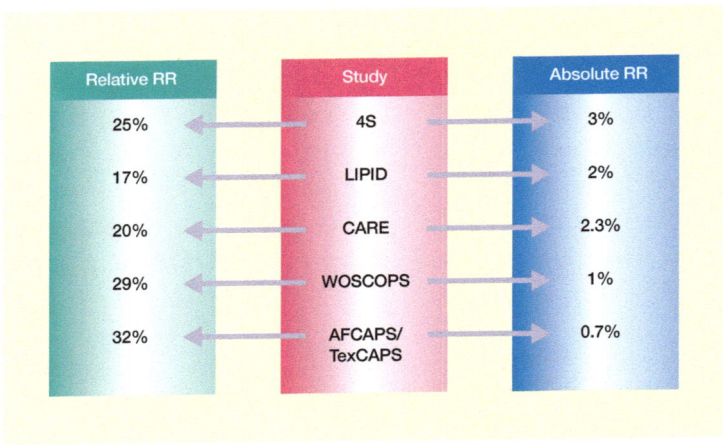

Relative RR	Study	Absolute RR
25%	4S	3%
17%	LIPID	2%
20%	CARE	2.3%
29%	WOSCOPS	1%
32%	AFCAPS/TexCAPS	0.7%

Figure 5.1   Absolute vs relative risk reductions in the major statin trials. Hazards are calculated on the most comprehensive endpoint per person-year and vary slightly between trials.

global risk. This has important implications for the number needed to treat (NNT) to prevent one event. This concept is an important one, which allows us to put risk reductions achieved with statins into a meaningful clinical context. For example, the NNT has been calculated to be 86 in the case of the low risk population studied in AFCAPS/TEXCAPS, while others have estimated the NNT in WOSCOPS, CARE and 4S to be approximately 43, 17 and 12, respectively. Clearly, the higher the risk the smaller the number of patients we need to treat to prevent one major event.

In order to make the most cost-effective use of statin therapy it is therefore important to assess the global risk of vascular disease in patients before deciding whether or not to treat. However, even if this approach is adopted, the question of what threshold risk level at which to treat remains. In many respects this question is not a medical one but a socio-economic one, in that the answer is determined by financial and health service considerations.

If the risk level for intervention with statins is set low then a large number of patients would be eligible for treatment, while a higher risk threshold would significantly reduce the number treated and the associated cost of therapy (Figure 5.2). Consequently, the threshold

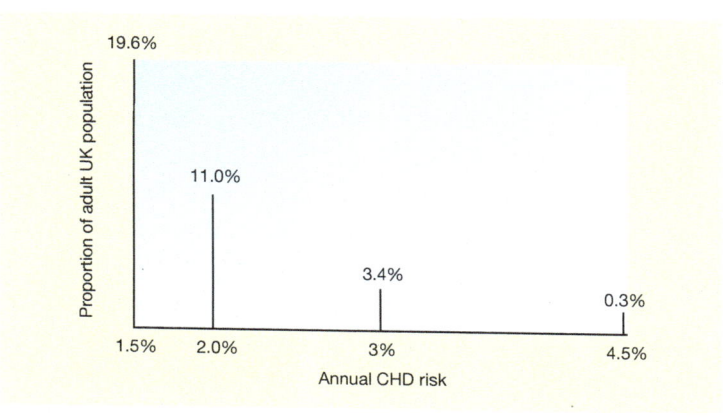

Figure 5.2   Proportions of the population that would be treated using different risk thresholds.

risk level that can be tolerated will vary from country to country and between different health care systems. Arguments for a 3% annual risk in primary prevention are put forward as a workable compromise between desirability and affordability and this level is advocated by the authors of the widely used Sheffield tables.

We would argue that the risk level chosen should at least encompass all patients who have suffered a vascular event, as the evidence for cost-effective protection with statins in these individuals is overwhelming. This approach of 'secondary prevention' is often viewed as distinct from the prevention or delay of first vascular events. So-called 'primary prevention' is viewed by many as a more controversial option, as it deals with patients at apparently much lower risk than those who have already demonstrated their high risk status by suffering an event. Furthermore, many view primary prevention as not being cost effective.

This is, to some extent, erroneous. First, a recent international cost-effectiveness analysis of the WOSCOPS study (a primary prevention study) has revealed that statin use is both clinically and cost-effective across a range of health care systems and the authors concluded that this primary prevention approach should fit within the bounds set by already accepted therapies in most countries. Second, as can be seen in Figure 5.3, the risk spectrum does not neatly separate 'primary' and 'secondary' prevention. Indeed, some individuals who have not yet suffered an event, such as the highest risk participants in WOSCOPS, actually have a higher global risk score than some of the post-myocardial infarction patients in CARE. Clearly, it is inappropriate to advocate 'secondary prevention' and simultaneously question the validity of higher risk 'primary prevention' if we believe in treating all patients at high risk.

Thus, the threshold risk level used should not only encompass all subjects who have suffered an event, but also those at highest risk of a first event. Any such level is, by necessity, arbitrary, but a figure of 2% per annum is both reasonable and one that was advocated by the original Joint European Guidelines. This argument

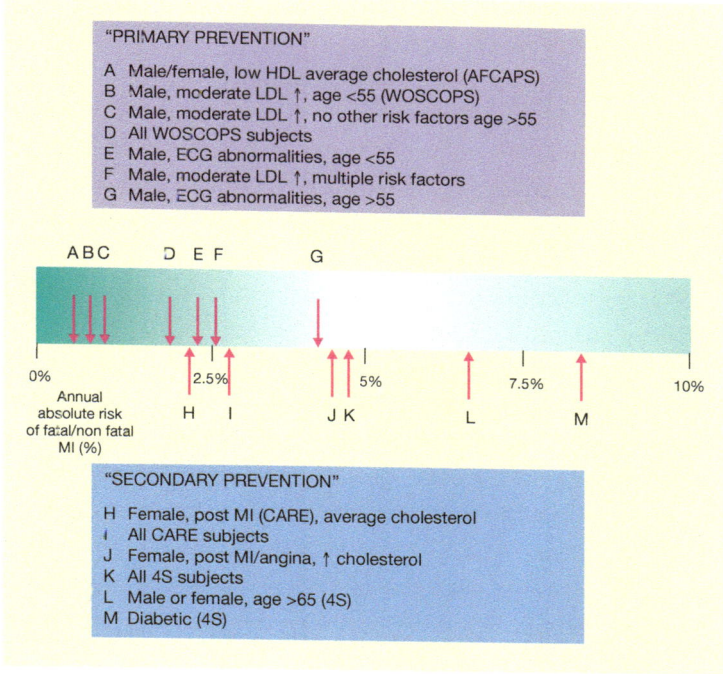

"PRIMARY PREVENTION"

A Male/female, low HDL average cholesterol (AFCAPS)
B Male, moderate LDL ↑, age <55 (WOSCOPS)
C Male, moderate LDL ↑, no other risk factors age >55
D All WOSCOPS subjects
E Male, ECG abnormalities, age <55
F Male, moderate LDL ↑, multiple risk factors
G Male, ECG abnormalities, age >55

A B C   D E F   G

0%   2.5%   5%   7.5%   10%
Annual
absolute risk   H I   J K   L   M
of fatal/non fatal
MI (%)

"SECONDARY PREVENTION"

H Female, post MI (CARE), average cholesterol
I All CARE subjects
J Female, post MI/angina, ↑ cholesterol
K All 4S subjects
L Male or female, age >65 (4S)
M Diabetic (4S)

Figure 5.3   CHD risk spectrum. The overlap between 'primary' and 'secondary' prevention is shown.

does, however, beg the question – how should global vascular risk be assessed?

Risk assessment

Statins, it may be argued should be prescribed, not on the basis of cholesterol levels alone, but rather using global risk scores that include lipid levels but do not depend on them. Others would support this argument against a lipocentric approach and indeed many guidelines outside the United States have taken this global risk approach.

There are a number of charts, calculators and computer programs available to assist the clinician. None of these devices is definitive, as none of them are able to incorporate all known CHD risk factors. For example, family history is often omitted from risk assessment tools despite the fact that this is regarded as one of the most important predictors of future vascular disease. However, all these tools serve to reduce the focus on single risk factors, in an attempt to assess the integrated or global risk. These relatively simple devices allow the clinician to combine a number of major discrete and continuous risk factors into a single risk score in the form of a percentage chance of suffering a major vascular event over the next 5–10 years, and then to base the treatment decision upon this number.

The choice of risk assessment tool has been the subject of some debate and a number of studies have compared different approaches. The revised Sheffield tables have recently been introduced, as have updated New Zealand tables. The new Sheffield tables incorporate a total cholesterol:HDL cholesterol ratio rather than total cholesterol alone in order to improve the accuracy of risk estimation. This has been one of the major criticisms of the former Sheffield tables, which some have regarded as significantly underestimating the risk in women. The New Zealand tables have proven popular since their introduction and a recent survey of the clinical usefulness of different risk assessment tools found that among doctors and nurses these tables were the most favoured, while the Sheffield tables were the least.

Whatever tool is used, it should be based on data derived from large prospective studies such as Framingham or PROCAM. The Framingham Heart Study risk equations have been shown to be valid in UK populations and these may be preferred. Also, with advancing technology it makes sense to adopt computerized or even interactive versions of these in order to maximize their utility. The most useful risk assessment devices are therefore likely to be computer based, Framingham derived, non-tabular systems, such as that accompanying the recently published Joint British Guidelines.

The practicalities of putting any risk assessment or treatment strategy into practice must also be considered alongside the scientific evidence that underpins it. Even with close clinical follow-up or detailed physician education it may be very difficult to achieve the implementation of any new set of guidelines.

Even accurate risk assessment, however, does not resolve all the challenges to the practising clinician in this field. Usually risk assessment is performed at baseline before intervention either by lifestyle approaches or by drug therapy. However, if risk assessment is repeated at a later date and as a result of lifestyle changes the risk estimate has fallen below the threshold for intervention, should drug therapy be ruled out?

Similarly, many physicians are perplexed by which risk factors they should tackle first in the high risk patient. Many patients will present with obesity, hypertension and hyperlipidaemia. This is a difficult situation but the clinician should adopt an evidence based approach and in doing so should intervene early, as appropriate, with statin therapy.

6 What about the future?

The growth of statin usage is almost exponential at present. In addition, new, even more powerful, statins are scheduled for launch in the next couple of years. Statins are being proposed for other therapeutic targets such as stroke and diabetes, but there remain many unanswered questions about the appropriate use of statins even in patients at risk of CHD. This section will take a forward look at these issues.

Unanswered questions

Despite the enormous amount of statin clinical trial data that has been assembled over the last decade there remain a number of clinically important questions to which we are only beginning to formulate answers. A number of these questions are being addressed in a series of large clinical trials that are currently underway. At present there are probably more than 30 major statin trials active, but it would not be possible to cover all of these here. Instead examples of these trials will be discussed in the context of the outstanding questions that they are attempting to answer.

Should statins be prescribed to the elderly?

The Prospective Study of Pravastatin in the Elderly at Risk (PROSPER) is a double-blind, randomized, placebo-controlled multi-centre study that was commenced in November 1997. It is designed to examine the hypothesis that pravastatin will reduce cardiovascular and cerebrovascular events in elderly subjects with either existing vascular disease or a high risk of developing the condition.

Approximately 5500 elderly men and women aged 70–82 years of age, with total plasma cholesterol of 4.0–9.0 mmol/l (155–348 mg/dl), triglyceride < 6 mmol/l (531 mg/dl) and good cognitive function were sought by community screening in the environs of Glasgow, Leiden and Cork.

Participants are randomized to 40 mg pravastatin/day or matching placebo, and are being followed up for a minimum of 3 years. The primary outcome measure is the combined endpoint of coronary heart disease (CHD) death (definite plus suspect), non-fatal MI (definite plus suspect) and fatal plus non-fatal stroke. Secondary analysis will examine the primary endpoint in each of the following subgroups: men, women, subjects with and without pre-existing stable angina, intermittent claudication, stroke, TIA, MI, arterial surgery and amputation for vascular disease.

Fatal plus non-fatal stroke and coronary events will also be reviewed separately as secondary endpoints, and tertiary outcomes will include disability, all cardiovascular events, vascular mortality, all cause mortality and cognitive function decline. The study is designed to include real-time assessments necessary for a health resource utilization and cost–benefit analysis that will be performed as a substudy to the protocol.

The project is currently under way in all three countries and patient recruitment was completed in April 1999 when 5804 subjects had been enrolled. The importance of the PROSPER study is its focus not only on stroke and TIA prevention in an elderly, at-risk population, but also on its efforts to test the hypothesis that statin therapy will prevent cognitive decline and preserve quality of life and independence in this group. It is also important to note that no distinction is drawn in this study between primary and secondary prevention, and that the lipid inclusion range is very wide. The results are expected in 2002.

Should statins be used in diabetes?

Type 2 diabetic patients are a very high risk group of patients with respect to vascular disease. Subgroup analysis from studies such as 4S and CARE has suggested that statin therapy would be even more effective in this group than in non-diabetic subjects. However, to date, no large scale intervention trials have been conducted specifically to address this question. This will change soon when the results of a series of statin and diabetes studies are published. An example of such a study is the CARDS (Collaborative Atorvastatin and Diabetes Study). This study of atorvastatin 10 mg versus placebo is being conducted in 2750 type 2 diabetics with no history of CHD but with one other CHD risk factor. The primary endpoint will be major cardiovascular events such as fatal and non-fatal MI, but will also include diabetic sequelae such as proteinuria and reinopathy.

Should statins be used to prevent stroke?

Again subgroup analyses from the large intervention trials with statins have provided some good evidence that simvastatin and pravastatin significantly reduce the rate of stroke in patients with pre-existing coronary disease. But what of stroke prevention in patients with no history of vascular disease or in those who have already suffered one or more cerebrovascular events? A number of major trials are under way to answer these questions. The large Heart Protection Study which has recruited more than 20 000 subjects includes a large number of stroke survivors. This placebo controlled study is examining the potential benefits of simvastatin and/or antioxidant vitamins in a 2 × 2 factorial design. Other large scale studies primarily looking at stroke include PROSPER described above and two others – SPARCL, a stroke secondary prevention study using atorvastatin, and RESPECT, an elderly stroke prevention study using cerivastatin.

Which statin is best?

Given that there are now six commercially available statins with five of these being currently marketed in the UK, this is an obvious and important clinical question. The statins are clearly not identical structurally or pharmacologically but the most important facet of their mechanism of action is their ability to prevent vascular events. Whether all statins are equal in this respect can only be tested in true head to head trials. A number of these are now under way. One of the largest is the PROVE IT study.

The PROVE IT (Pravastatin or Atorvastatin Evaluation and Infection Therapy) trial was announced at the end of 1999 and will be the first head to head trial to compare pravastatin and atorvastatin, using a clinical event endpoint. This clinical trial is also designed to study the effects of anti-infective therapy (gatifloxacin) on cardiovascular event reduction with regard to the role of *Chlamydia pneumoniae*. In addition, PROVE IT will measure inflammatory markers of coronary heart disease, including C-reactive protein.

The PROVE IT trial is a double blind, randomized trial that will enrol approximately 4000 patients, at 500 US and international sites, who have experienced an acute coronary syndrome within the previous 10 days. Patients will receive either 40 mg of pravastatin or 80 mg of atorvastatin shortly following their event and will be followed for a period of at least 1.5 years. The primary endpoint of the trial will be a composite of major cardiovascular events.

To study the role of infection in CHD, one half of the patients in the trial will also receive the antibiotic gatifloxacin in addition to either statin. The other half of the patient population will receive an antibiotic placebo (a 2×2 factorial randomization).

New lipid lowering strategies

The clinical benefits of statins are so impressive that some enthusiasts have been emboldened to write that they 'are to atherosclerosis what penicillin was to infectious disease'. Taking that analogy one step further might lead us to wonder whether statins represent the pinnacles of our needs as far as lipid lowering is concerned. If antibiotics have taught us anything it must surely be that complacency is dangerous.

Cholesterol lowering with statin therapy might not be the whole answer to atherosclerosis and vascular disease prevention, for it may be argued that if it were, coronary events would have been eliminated in the published trials rather than 'merely' reduced by 30%. Clinical trials are of course not the whole story and do not systematically test the multiple risk factor modification approach that should be adopted in daily clinical practice.

However, there is another more cogent reason why we should gain comfort from continuing lipid lowering drug development. The primary mechanism of action of statins is to promote the clearance of LDL from the circulation. But the majority of dyslipidaemic patients admitted to the coronary care unit usually exhibit raised plasma cholesterol and triglyceride levels rather than hypercholesterolaemia alone. While the statins were specifically designed to deal with the latter problem, their ability to lower plasma triglyceride levels is usually more limited.

Thus, the pharmaceutical industry has embarked on a search for new drugs to target triglyceride rich lipoprotein production and some of these drugs are currently in early trials. One other approach to lipid lowering that may complement statin therapy is the development of drugs to block cholesterol absorption from the gut, while yet another is to seek new drugs that will act primarily on raising HDL cholesterol. There is certainly no shortage of activity in this rapidly evolving field and we can expect several novel lipid lowering drugs in the next decade.

Improving patient compliance

As with any chronic medication for an asymptomatic condition, statin therapy is unfortunately associated with relatively poor patient compliance. Indeed some investigators report a 50% drop-out rate from therapy after only 12 months. Impressive as the clinical trial results may be with statin therapy we will never translate these findings into clinical reality if we cannot achieve better compliance amongst our patients. In order to assist us in this goal it is worthwhile examining the background to our patients' and our own perceptions of CHD risk. These have recently been evaluated in a series of surveys.

Patients perceive a greater risk of CHD from smoking and parental death from a coronary event than from cholesterol and blood pressure. In a primary care survey of middle-aged men and women, more patients were optimistic (37%) than pessimistic (21%) about their risk of developing CHD. Over-optimistic perceptions of risk and indifferent attitudes to change may explain why health promotion campaigns have had only a modest effect in changing attitudes about prevention of CHD.

Even post-MI patients have been reported to be more concerned about the risks of non-cardiovascular diseases. The recent pan-European HELP study was designed to provide more information about awareness and attitudes towards reducing CHD. The investigators interviewed over 10 000 patients across Europe. This study found that individuals had a reasonable knowledge of the risks involved in triggering an acute coronary event, yet many displayed an indifference to reducing this risk, even those who had suffered a previous MI.

Both the general public and high risk groups identified cancer and heart disease as the two major causes of death. Surprisingly, 72% of the general public claimed to have had their cholesterol checked, compared with only 51% of the high risk group. However, more patients in both of these groups said they had received information about cholesterol reduction from friends and magazines rather than from their doctor. Despite this, both groups rated the cardiologist, primary-care physician and hospital as the three most credible sources of information.

Although post-MI patients said that they were not overly worried about experiencing another heart attack, 80% reported making spontaneous changes to their lifestyle after the heart attack. More post-MI patients received information from the medical profession than from television, magazines and newspapers, compared with the general public (Table 6.1). However, only 23% of the post-MI group had been warned that their cholesterol level was too high and, of these patients, only 21% could recall their cholesterol level, while 16% of the post-MI patients reported being advised to lower their blood

Table 6.1   Proportion of the general public and post-MI patients who obtain their heart health information from healthcare professionals and from various media sources (adapted from Shepherd et al, 1999).

Source	Percentage (%) of patients	
	General public	**Post-MI patients**
Television	20	5
Newspapers	18	4
Magazines	14	2
Doctor	16	30
Cardiologist	2	28
Consultant	2	13
Family	6	2
Friends	5	1
Don't know	6	3
Other	11	12

pressure. Of the post-MI group, 53% claimed to have followed all of their primary-care physician's advice, while 27% reported to have followed most of it. All groups also returned a very high level of satisfaction with the advice given by the primary-care physician.

The HELP study concluded that although patients had access to many sources of heart health information, which in the case of the medical profession were perceived as highly credible, this had only a limited impact on their adherence to preventive treatments and advice. This study also highlights the fact that once information is provided, little is done to ensure it is implemented. It seems that where lifestyle changes fail to be carried through, the use of statin therapy is less than adequate. In post-MI patients, in particular, the medical profession believes that only certain messages such as diet, exercise, smoking, regular screening and stress management are getting through to patients, whereas messages of cholesterol lowering, therapy compliance, weight reduction and family screening are not (Table 6.2).

Table 6.2   Physicians' perceptions about which messages regarding CHD prevention are succeeding and which are failing to get through to post-MI patients (adapted from Shepherd et al, 1999).

Succeeding	Failing
Diet and health	Cholesterol lowering
Exercise	Therapy compliance
Smoking	Weight reduction
Regular screening	Family screening
Stress management	

Barriers to implementing statin therapy

We now know what we should be doing but often it does not happen. Why should this be so? Many barriers have been identified which obstruct the implementation of evidence-based therapy in the secondary prevention of CHD. This treatment gap may result from one or more weaknesses in the chain of responsibilities to provide risk-reduction care. These include the formulation and implementation of a risk-reduction plan by the hospital, the effectiveness with which the plan is communicated to primary-care follow-up, the formulation of a new plan or implementation of the hospital-recommended plan and finally patient compliance with the treatment plan.

Primary-care physicians and their nurses are in a favourable position to take on the task of secondary CHD prevention because they have an ongoing relationship with the patient, which offers them the chance to monitor the patient's progress, motivate the patient to make lifestyle changes and ensure long term compliance with drug therapy.

The lack of clear, national or local guidelines for secondary prevention is reported to be a shared barrier for both cardiologists and primary-care physicians in taking any preventive action. However, in England at least this may now be dealt with in the form of the recently published National Service Framework for Coronary Heart Disease.

Here, despite its many critics is a reasonable attempt at formulating a national and consistent strategy. Embedded in this strategy is a firm and unequivocal endorsement of statin use both in primary and secondary prevention.

Statin prescribing tomorrow

Despite all the difficulties, the appropriate prescription of statin therapy is growing rapidly, stimulated no doubt by the publication of new and authoritative evidence-based guidelines. The one remaining barrier to full implementation is financial. Many economists, health professionals and governments remain concerned over the impact that this will have on healthcare budgets. Consequently, old, unproven, albeit cheaper therapeutic approaches remain in place despite evidence of the clear benefits of statin therapy. This is poor medicine and of questionable benefit to society. However, the weight of clinical trial evidence is now so strong that it is impossible to ignore and new strategy documents produced by traditionally conservative bodies now firmly endorse the appropriate use of statins in both primary and secondary prevention.

These cost-containment arguments will, however, dissolve in the future as the loss of statin patent protection, which will occur over the next few years, will lead to the introduction of lower priced statin generics. Indeed, in the foreseeable future, and subject to the longer term proven safety of these drugs, statins may receive widespread over-the-counter status, thereby transferring the cost consideration of their use from health authorities to the individual. Perhaps then, evidence based medicine will truly be adopted.

Glossary of terms

Apolipoproteins, these are special proteins that are present in lipoproteins. They are named by letters and numbers and each has a specific structural or metabolic function.

Apo A-I, apolipoprotein A-I, is the major apolipoprotein in HDL.

Apo B, apolipoprotein B is the major apolipoprotein of VLDL, IDL and LDL and acts as a ligand for the LDL receptor.

Apo C-II apolipoprotein C-II is the cofactor necessary for the action of lipoprotein lipase.

Apo E, apolipoprotein E is present in VLDL, HDL and chylomicron remnants and acts as a ligand for the LDL receptor.

Arcus, *see* Corneal arcus.

Arteriosclerosis, means hardening of the arteries. This term is often used interchangeably with atherosclerosis but it is a much less specific term describing a broad range of vascular pathology.

Atheroma, *see* Atherosclerosis.

Atherosclerosis, a chronic disease process characterized by a focal, inflammatory fibro-proliferative response to multiple forms of endothelial injury. This results in the build-up of fibro-fatty deposits called plaques within the artery wall.

Atorvastatin, an HMG CoA reducatse inhibitor that is unique in having a prolonged half-life. This statin was used in the AVERT and MIRACL trials.

Beta-quantification, form of lipid profiling that provides the following measurements: total cholesterol, total triglyceride, LDL cholesterol, VLDL cholesterol and HDL cholesterol.

Bezafibrate, a fibric acid derivative used in the management of patients with dyslipidaemia; principally those with hypertriglyceridaemia and low HDL.

Bile acid sequestrant resin, class of lipid lowering drugs. These compounds are not absorbed from the gut but bind bile acids and prevent their reabsorption from the terminal ileum. The liver has then to increase its synthesis of bile acids which it does by using the circulating cholesterol as a building block. These drugs therefore result in lowering of plasma cholesterol and more specifically the LDL cholesterol.

BMI, *see* body mass index.

Body mass index, calculated by dividing the body weight in kilogrammes by the height squared in metres.

CAD, *see* coronary artery disease.

Cerivastatin, an HMG CoA reductase inhibitor or statin prescribed in microgramme rather than milligramme doses.

CETP, *see* Cholesteryl ester transfer protein.

CHD, *see* Coronary heart disease.

Cholesterol, a white waxy substance insoluble in water. Cholesterol is composed of 27 carbon atoms in the form of four interconnecting rings with a tail. It is found only in animal cells; plants cannot manufacture cholesterol.

Cholesteryl ester, form of cholesterol in which a fatty acid is attached to its third carbon through an ester bond. This is the storage form of cholesterol which is found inside cells and in the core of lipoproteins.

Cholesteryl ester transfer protein, an enzyme involved in the exchange of cholesteryl esters and triglyceride between lipoproteins.

Cholestyramine, a bile acid sequestrant resin used in the treatment of hypercholesterolaemia.

Chylomicron, the largest of the lipoproteins, this particle is made in the gut where it is used to carry fats from the diet to the rest of the body. It is normally absent from the bloodstream after an overnight fast.

Ciprofibrate, a fibric acid derivative used in the management of patients with dyslipidaemia; principally those with hypertr glyceridaemia and low HDL.

Colestipol, a bile acid sequestrant resin used in the treatment of hypercholesterolaemia.

Corneal arcus, deposit of cholesterol in the clear outer covering (cornea) of the eye. Corneal arcus before the age of about 55 years is usually indicative of an underlying lipid disorder. However, when present in the elderly (arcus senilis) it does not have the same significance.

Coronary arteries, the arteries that supply blood and therefore oxygen and nutrients to the heart muscle. There are three major coronary arteries: the right coronary artery, the left anterior descending coronary artery and the left circumflex coronary artery.

Coronary artery disease, see Coronary heart disease.

Coronary heart disease, this is the commonest cause of serious illness and death in the Western world. It results from blockages of the coronary arteries and leads to the development of angina if the blockages are incomplete or a myocardial infarction if the coronary arteries become completely occluded.

Dyslipidaemia, any disorder characterized by an aberrant lipid profile often used when a general term is required to cover both increased lipid levels, abnormal patterns and decreased lipid levels.

Endothelium, the layer of cells that line the interior surface of any blood vessel.

Familial combined hyperlipidaemia (FCH), an inherited disorder causing premature coronary heart disease in which affected individuals have either a raised blood cholesterol level alone, a raised blood triglyceride level alone or both.

Familial hypercholesterolaemia (FH), an inherited disorder causing premature coronary heart disease in which affected individuals have high levels of total cholesterol and specifically LDL cholesterol. FH is due to an inherited defect in the LDL receptor that prevents removal of LDL particles from the bloodstream at a normal rate. Subjects with a single faulty copy of the LDL receptor gene are called FH heterozygotes and those with two faulty copies are called FH homozygotes.

Fasting sample, a blood sample collected after a 12–14 hour fast (i.e. no foods or calorie containing fluids consumed). This is done to obtain a lipid profile 'uncontaminated' by dietary lipids.

Fatty acid, a member of the lipid family, this type of molecule consists of a chain of carbon atoms whose length and degree of saturation vary. Saturated fatty acids are those where all the positions in the carbon chain are occupied or saturated with hydrogen atoms. A monounsaturated fatty acid is one where a single position in the carbon chain is unsaturated, i.e. two adjacent carbon atoms are missing one hydrogen atom.

Fatty streak, the earliest visible stage of the atherosclerotic process. These are slightly raised yellow streaks visible on the interior of the artery and are due to the accumulation of lipid filled macrophages within the artery wall.

FCH, *see* Familial combined hyperlipidaemia.

Fenofibrate, a fibric acid derivative used in the management of patients with dyslipidaemia, principally those with hypertriglyceridaemia and low HDL.

FH, *see* Familial hypercholesterolaemia.

Fibrate, a drug derived from fibric acid used to lower blood lipid levels (*see also* Fenofibrate, Ciprofibrate, Gemfibrozil).

Fluvastatin, the first synthetic HMG CoA reductase inhibitor.

Fredrickson's classification, the WHO classification of lipid disorders which is based on a phenotypic analysis of the plasma appearance and the lipid levels. This system divides lipid disorders into six classes: types I, IIa, IIb, III, IV and V hyperlipoproteinaemia.

Gemfibrozil, a fibric acid derivative used in the management of patients with dyslipidaemia; principally those with hypertriglyceridaemia and low HDL.

HDL, *see* High density lipoprotein.

Heterozygote, an individual with two different copies of a gene, usually one normal and one faulty.

High density lipoprotein (HDL), a lipoprotein that carries about 20–25% of the blood cholesterol. About 50% of HDL is protein, the major constituent being apoA-I. HDL removes cholesterol from the surface of cells, esterifies it and then transfers the cholesteryl ester to other lipoproteins for delivery to the liver for processing. HDL is sometimes referred to as 'good' cholesterol because high levels of HDL are associated with a lower risk of coronary heart disease and low levels with higher risk.

HMG CoA reductase inhibitor, a class of drugs also known as statins that block the manufacture of cholesterol by cells by inhibiting the action of the enzyme HMG CoA reductase. These drugs reduce the amount of cholesterol inside cells, leading to an increase in the number of LDL receptors on the cell surface and increased removal of LDL from the blood.

Homozygote, an individual with two identical copies of a gene, usually both faulty.

Hypercholesterolaemia, a high level of total cholesterol in the blood.

Hyperlipidaemia, a high level of lipids (cholesterol, triglyceride or both) in the blood.

Hypertriglyceridaemia, a high level of total triglyceride in the blood.

IDL, *see* Intermediate density lipoprotein.

Intermediate density lipoprotein (IDL), a transient intermediate generated from VLDL en route to LDL as a byproduct of the breakdown of triglyceride in VLDL and VLDL remnants. IDL is relatively enriched in cholesterol. Some IDL is removed from the bloodstream by the LDL receptor and the remainder is converted to LDL by further delipidation.

Ischaemia, lack of oxygen to cells, leading to injury and, if severe enough, to permanent damage or scarring of the tissue.

Joint European Guidelines, Recommendations of the European Society of Cardiology, European Atherosclerosis Society and European Society of Hypertension. This is an important consensus statement by three large European organizations and includes detailed guidelines for the screening and treatment of individuals at risk of coronary disease.

LDL, *see* Low density lipoprotein.

LDL receptor, a cell surface receptor present on many cell types that is involved in the trapping and internalization of lipoprotein particles, mainly LDL and IDL. This receptor was discovered by Joseph Goldstein and Michael Brown who won the Nobel Prize in 1985 for their work. Defects in the LDL receptor result in the condition familial hypercholesterolaemia.

Lipid, any substance that is insoluble in water but soluble in apolar solvents, such as ether or chloroform.

Lipid clinic, usually hospital based this is a clinic that specializes in the diagnosis and management of dyslipidaemias.

Lipid profile, a blood test in which the blood levels of cholesterol, triglyceride and some combination of HDL, VLDL and LDL cholesterol are measured.

Lipoprotein, a complex of proteins called apolipoproteins and lipids, such as cholesterol, cholesteryl esters, triglyceride and phospholipids. Lipoproteins are responsible for transporting lipids between various organs of the body.

Lipoprotein lipase, an enzyme that is responsible for the breakdown of triglyceride in either chylomicrons or VLDL.

Lovastatin, the first HMG CoA reductase inhibitor to reach clinical practice.

Low density lipoprotein (LDL), is the major carrier of cholesterol in blood. A high level of LDL promotes the development of atherosclerosis and, in turn, coronary heart disease.

Macrophage, a scavenger cell that is involved in many of the protective inflammatory responses in the body and which has a key role in the development of the atherosclerotic plaque.

Monounsaturated fats, clear oily substances that are liquid at room temperature. Monounsaturated fats (e.g. olive oil) are rich in monounsaturated fatty acids.

Myocardial infarction, when the muscle of the heart (myocardium) is deprived of oxygen the muscle cells die (infarction). This process is often called a heart attack. If the patient survives the infarcted area will heal but will remain scarred.

Phospholipids, a class of lipids usually containing a glycerol backbone, two fatty acids and a third polar component in which a chemical compound is attached to the glycerol through its phosphorus component. Phospholipids act as detergent molecules.

Plaque, *see* Atherosclerosis.

Polyunsaturated fats, clear oily substances that are liquid at room temperature. Polyunsaturated fats (e.g. safflower and sunflower oils) are rich in polyunsaturated fatty acids.

Post-prandial lipaemia, the increase in blood lipid levels seen after a meal.

Pravastatin, an HMG CoA reductase inhibitor used in the West of Scotland Study Coronary Prevention Study, the CARE study and the LIPID trial.

Primary prevention, as applied to coronary prevention this term is used to describe the strategy of preventing coronary events from occurring in normal, healthy individuals.

Regression, the process whereby atheromatous plaques shrink in size as a result of aggressive lipid lowering therapy.

Resin, *see* Bile acid sequestrant resin; Cholestyramine; Colestipol.

Rhabdomyolysis, destruction of the skeletal muscle which leads to kidney failure. This is a rare but potentially serious side effect of statin therapy.

Risk factor, as applied to atherosclerosis, a condition or state that predisposes to the development and progression of atherosclerosis. The major risk factors are male gender, smoking, dyslipidaemia, hypertension, diabetes, obesity and family history of premature coronary heart disease. The evidence for these comes primarily from the large and still ongoing epidemiological survey of cardiovascular disease, the Framingham Study, and from the Multiple Risk Factor Intervention Trial (MRFIT).

Saturated fats, white, oily substances that are solid at room temperature. Chemically, these fats are esters of glycerol and saturated fatty acids. Saturated fats are the main constituent of the visible fat around meat, of butter and cheese, and of whole milk and ice-cream. Saturated fats are also plentiful in coconut oil, palm kernel oil and palm oil, three vegetable oils widely used in commercially processed foods.

Secondary prevention, as applied to coronary prevention this term is used to describe the strategy of preventing further coronary events in patients who have already been diagnosed as having angina or peripheral vascular disease, or who have suffered a myocardial infarction.

Simvastatin, an HMG CoA reductase inhibitor that was used in the 4S (Scandinavian Simvastatin Survival Study) trial, the first secondary prevention trial to show that lipid lowering can save lives.

Statin, *see* HMG CoA reductase inhibitor; Atorvastatin; Cerivastatin; Fluvastatin; Lovastatin; Pravastatin; Simvastatin.

Triglyceride, also called triacylglycerol, a member of the lipid family in which three fatty acids are attached to a glycerol backbone through ester bonds.

Very low density lipoprotein (VLDL), is the major carrier of triglyceride in the bloodstream of the fasting subject. VLDL is assembled in the liver and contains about 65% of its weight as triglyceride. It also contains apo B, apo E and apo C. As the triglyceride in VLDL is broken down by the action of lipoprotein lipase, VLDL remnants and then IDL are produced. Some of these particles are taken up by the liver via its cell surface receptors, but the rest are converted into LDL.

VLDL, *see* Very low density lipoprotein.

Xanthelasma, yellowish, flat deposits of lipid on the eyelids or under the eyes often indicating the presence of a dyslipidaemia

Xanthoma, a deposit of lipid in the skin or tendons. Xanthomas occur in people with several different kinds of blood lipid disorders. Achilles and elbow tendon xanthomas are particularly common in people with FH.

Further reading

Brown MS, Goldstein JL (1987) The LDL receptor. In: Gallo LL, ed, *Cardiovascular Disease* (Plenum Press: New York) 87–91.

Campbell NC, Thain J, Deans HG et al (1998) Secondary prevention in coronary heart disease: baseline survey of provision in general practice, *Br Med J* **326**:1430–4.

Caro J, Klittich W, McGuire A et al (1999) International economic analysis of primary prevention of cardiovascular disease with pravastatin in WOSCOPS, *Eur Heart J* **20**:263–8.

Downs JR, Clearfield M, Weis S et al (1998) Primary prevention of acute coronary events with lovastatin in men and women with average cholesterol levels: results of AFCAPS/TEXCAPS Research Group, *JAMA* **279**:1615–22.

Durrington PN, Prais H, Bhatnagar D et al (1999) Indications for cholesterol-lowering medication: comparison of risk-assessment methods, *Lancet* **353**:278–81.

EUROASPIRE study group (1997) A European Society of Cardiology survey on secondary prevention of coronary heart disease: principal results, *Eur Heart J* **18**:1569–82.

Falk E, Shah PK, Fuster V. (1995) Coronary plaque disruption, *Circulation* **92**:657–71.

Gaw A, Cowan RA, O'Reilly D St J (1995) Clinical biochemistry: an illustrated colour text, Churchill Livingstone, Edinburgh.

Gaw A, Packard CJ, Shepherd J (eds) (2000) *Statins. The HMG CoA Reductase Inhibitors in Perspective* (Martin Dunitz, London).

Grover SA, Lowensteyn I, Esrey KL et al (1995) Do doctors accurately assess coronary risk in their patients? Preliminary results of the coronary health assessment study, *Br Med J* **310**:975–8.

Grundy SM (1986) Cholesterol and heart disease: a new era, *JAMA* **256**:2849–58.

Grundy SM. (1999) Primary prevention of coronary heart disease. Integrating risk assessment with intervention, *Circulation* **100**: 988–98.

Hingorami AD, Vallance P (1999) A simple computer program for guiding management of cardiovascular risk factors and prescribing, *Br Med J* **318**:101–5.

Hulscher MEJL, van Drenth BB, Mokkink HGA et al (1997) Effects of outreach visits by trained nurses on cardiovascular risk-factor recording in general practice: a controlled trial, *Eur J Gen Pract* **3**:90–5.

Isles CG, Ritchie LD, Murchie P, Norrie J (2000) Risk assessment in primary prevention of coronary heart disease: randomised comparison of three scoring methods, *Br Med J* **320**:690–1.

Jackson R (2000) Updated New Zealand cardiovascular disease risk–benefit prediction guide. *Br Med J* **320**:709–10.

Kannel WB, Castelli W, Gordon T et al (1971) Serum cholesterol lipoproteins and risk of coronary heart disease: the Framingham Study, *Ann Intern Med* **74**:1–12.

Keys, A (1980) *Seven Countries: A Multivariate Analysis of Death and Coronary Heart Disease* (Harvard University Press: Cambridge, MA).

Kleinveld HA, Demacker PNM, de Haan AFJ, Stalenhoef AFH (1993) Decreased in vitro oxidisability of LDL in hypercholesterolemic patients treated with HMG CoA reductase inhibitors, *Eur J Clin Invest* **23**:289–95.

Kobashigawa J, Katznelson S, Laks H et al (1995) Effect of pravastatin on outcomes after cardiac transplantation, *N Engl J Med* **333**:621–7.

Lacoste L, Lam JYT, Hung J et al (1995) Hyperlipidemia and coronary disease: correction of the increased thrombogenic potential with cholesterol reduction, *Circulation* **92**:3172–7.

LIPID Study Group (1998) Prevention of cardiovascular events and death with pravastatin in patients with coronary heart disease and a broad range of cholesterol levels, *N Engl J Med* **339**:1349–57.

Marmot MG, Syme SL, Kagan A et al (1975) Epidemiologic studies of coronary heart disease and stroke in Japanese men living in Japan, Hawaii and California: prevalence of coronary and hypertensive heart disease and associated risk factors, *Am J Epidemiol* **102**:514–25.

Marteau TM, Kinmonth AI, Pyke S, Thompson SG (1995) Readiness for lifestyle advice: self-assessments of coronary risk prior to screening in the British Family Heart Study. Family Heart Study Group, *Br J Gen Pract* **45**:3905–8.

Martin MJ, Hulley SB, Browner WS et al (1986) Serum cholesterol, blood pressure and mortality: implications from a cohort of 361 662 men, *Lancet* **2**: 933–6.

National Service Framework for Coronary Heart Disease. London: Dept of Health, 2000.

Pickin DM, McCabe CJ, Ramsey LE et al (1999) Cost effectiveness of HMG-CoA reductase inhibitor (statin) treatment related to the risk of coronary heart disease and cost of drug treatment, *Heart* **82**:325–32.

Poulter N, Sever P, Thom S (1993) Cardiovascular disease: practical issues for prevention. Caroline Black, St Albans.

Pyörälä K, De Backer G, Graham I, Poole-Wilson P, Wood D (1994) Prevention of coronary heart disease in clinical practice. Recommendations of the Task Force of the European Society of Cardiology, European Atherosclerosis Society and European Society of Hypertension, *Eur Heart J* **15**:1300–31.

Ramachandran S, French JM, Vanderpump MPJ, Croft P, Neary RH (2000) Using the Framingham model to predict heart disease in the United Kingdom: retrospective study, *Br Med J* **320**:676–7.

Ributs WC (1996) The underused miracle: the statin drugs are to atherosclerosis what penicillin was to infectious disease, *Am J Cardiol* **78**:377–8.

Ridker PM, Cushman M, Stampfer MJ, Tracey RP, Hennekens CH (1997) Inflammation, aspirin, and the risk of cardiovascular disease in apparently healthy men, *N Engl J Med* **336**:973–9.

Rumley A. Lower GDO, Norrie J et al (1997) Blood rheology and outcome in the West of Scotland Coronary Prevention Study, *Br J Haematol* **97**:78(Abstr).

Sacks FM, Pfeffer MA, Moye LA et al (1996) The effect of pravastatin on coronary events after myocardial infarction in patients with average cholesterol levels, *N Engl J Med* **335**:1001–9.

Scandinavian Simvastatin Survival Study Group (1994). Randomised trial of cholesterol lowering in 4444 patients with coronary heart disease: The Scandinavian Simvastatin Survival Study (4S), *Lancet* **344**:1383–9.

Shepherd J, Blauw GJ, Murphy MB et al (1999) The design of a prospective study of pravastatin in the elderly at risk (PROSPER), *Am J Cardiol* **84**:1192–7.

Shepherd J, Cobbe SM, Ford I et al (1995) Prevention of coronary heart disease with pravastatin in men with hypercholesterolemia, *N Engl J Med* **333**:1301–7.

Simons LA (1986) Interrelations of lipids and lipoproteins with coronary artery disease mortality in 19 countries, *Am J Cardiol* **57**: Suppl G 5–10.

Soma MR, Parolini C, Donetti E et al (1995) Inhibition of isoprenoid biosynthesis and arterial smooth muscle cell proliferation, *J Cardiovasc Pharm* **25**(Suppl 4):S20–S24.

Standing medical advisory committee on the use of statins. NSH Executive (1997) (Department of Health: London).

Wallis EJ, Ramsay LE, Haq IU et al (2000) Coronary and cardiovascular risk estimation for primary prevention: validation of a new Sheffield table in the 1995 Scottish health survey population, *Br Med J* **320**:671–6.

West of Scotland Coronary Prevention Study Group (1998) Influence of pravastatin and plasma lipids on clinical events in the West of Scotland Coronary Prevention Study (WOSCOPS), *Circulation* **97**:1440–5.

Wood DA, De Backer G, Faergeman O et al (1998) Prevention of coronary heart disease in clinical practice. Recommendation of the second joint task force of the European Society of Cardiology, European Atherosclerosis Society and European Society of Hypertension, *Eur Heart J* **19**:1434–503

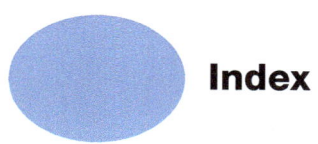

Index

Note: References to figures are indicated by 'f' and references to tables by 't' when they fall on a page not covered by the text reference.